Dr. Amarnick's

Mind Over Matter Pain Relief Program

Claude Amarnick, D.O.

A psychiatrist and rehabilitation specialist
confronts the chronic pain of body, mind and spirit.

Published by Garrett Publishing, Inc.
384 S. Military Trail
Deerfield Beach, Florida 33442
All rights reserved
©1995 Claude Amarnick

Library of Congress Catalog Card Number 95-081679
Dr. Claude Amarnick, D.O.
Dr. Amarnick's Mind Over Matter Pain Relief Program
Deerfield Beach, Florida
220 pages
ISBN 1-880539-36-5:$9.95

Cover design by Lloyd MacDonald.

Acknowledgements

This book would not have happened without the professional know-how and, when needed, the shirtsleeves hard work of Dr. Arnold Goldstein. Editor Candice Richard honed the words of a prolific writer. From manuscript to marketing, this book reflects the much-appreciated efforts of Ginny Holm, Joanne Milelli, and Beverly Sanders. Thanks also to the doctors and others in the field of medicine, here and abroad, whose encouragement before and after this book was written helped fulfill a dream.

Imagine that you can create the kind of life you want to live by believing you are already living it.

Table of Contents

Foreword

Millions of Americans suffer chronic pain. If you are one of them, this book will give you control over your pain so you can regain control over your life and look forward to a pain-free future.

Chronic pain affects your entire being: body, mind and spirit. You cannot treat the pain while ignoring the person. In this book I will show you the crucial links between mind-body-spirit. Chronic pain sufferers who do not understand the importance of this connection are victimized by the vicious cycle and spiraling effect of chronic pain—which is why only a holistic approach to chronic pain can succeed. That is the premise of this book.

Pain Relief provides a unique overview of Jungian philosophy, the Eastern belief connecting the inner self and the effect of the mind on physical pain. I explain the pain-destroying powers of yoga, T'ai Chi Chuan, creative visualization, guided imagery and meditation. I provide comprehensive case histories to reveal the benefits of my proven pain control process.

Unique to this book is Chapter 10, which discusses how childhood abuse relates to chronic pelvic pain. As emphasized in this chapter and throughout the book, forgiving oneself and others enables the chronic pain sufferer to manage the daily events of his or her life without the burdens of chronic pain. That is also the goal of this book.

Dr. Amarnick's chronic pain management program

I originally developed my multi-disciplinary pain-solving approach at my rehabilitation medical center in Queens, New York. With my staff of physical and occupational therapists, vocational rehabilitation counselors, psychologists and social workers, I formulated a comprehensive program to help patients control pain. That it worked so well in this conservative, multi-ethnic, middle-class neighborhood convinced me that this program did not require a psychologically sophisticated audience. It could be used successfully throughout the country. In fact, it has since been adopted by similar centers in Florida and California.

These pain centers represent the last resort for hundreds of desperate chronic pain patients and their families. They offer intensive interdisciplinary therapy, starting with an in-depth physical and psychological assessment of the patient's needs. Based on that evaluation, patients, families and staff collaborate to design a personal treatment program. The objective is for the individual to transcend the pain and learn new ways to control it.

Patients at these centers progress from passive forms of physical therapy to active strengthening and range of motion exercises. These activities are supplemented with relaxation techniques, creative visualization, meditation and imaging. You can include any or all of these activities in your own personalized program.

While many of these activities can be performed at home, there are some activities best performed in a more formal setting, such as a pain center with certified physical and occupational therapists, social workers with family-systems experience, or a psychologist.

Transcending chronic pain means focusing less on attaining relief and more on maintaining a calm composure and retaining self-respect. This will give you dignity, purpose and joy in life—despite the pain. Most Eastern religions consider pain an ephemeral experience: Only the mind or soul is real. Pain—like all bodily feelings—can be transcended. As Eastern thought believes, if pain has any meaning, it is as a guide to spiritual evolution.

Pain Relief is a valuable tool to shape your own pain management program, even if, like most chronic pain patients, you live miles from the nearest hospital or pain center. You can use my do-it-yourself techniques as well as the suggested resources available in your community. Pain sufferers need a nearby support system, not one thousands of miles away. Combining the family system with the pain control process, you can apply clearly laid out principles at home.

The goals

The goals in the pain management process, then, are threefold:

1. To rehabilitate rather than cure. That is, you learn to control rather than abolish pain and its effects.

2. To increase your functional activities.

3. To reduce your "illness behavior."

A typical program combines:

- exercise

- medication reduction

- relaxation techniques

- creative visualization

- meditation

- physical and occupational therapy

- behavior modification

- individual, group and family therapy.

A pain management program will enable you to increase your strength, mobility and the scope of your activities without drugs or other unnecessary aids.

Detach yourself from the pain. When you do, you no longer feel isolated from colleagues, family and friends. You no longer view treatment as a matter of straightening out a few nuts and bolts gone awry. The daily practice of creative visualization and meditation shifts consciousness—from identifying with the body and its pain to witnessing the pain to transcending the pain. If you can detach yourself from your pain, you can adapt to it.

As you gain a clearer sense of who you are, you will interact more successfully with others. Heightening your perception by engaging in spiritual practices allows you to fully realize your sense of self. Best of all, you learn to take care of yourself. Control increases as your physical condition, attitude and ability to take care of yourself improve.

Because of pain's far-reaching effects, my book encourages you and your family to examine all aspects of your lives. It aims to transform not only your physical condition, but how pain affects how you and those close to you think, feel and behave.

You can do the most important aspects of my program—physical exercise, creative visualization and meditation—on your own. You alone transcend the pain. I also help you find the community resources pain patients need, and reveal how to reduce your medications under your doctor's care. These points come alive through case histories of patients' lives that demonstrate how their transformations came about. So too will yours!

Chronic pain may be the symbolic physical expression of otherwise repressed feelings. Images of ourselves formed in our early years often shape feelings and behaviors later in life. Chronic pain symptoms can be a manifestation of inner conflict—perhaps an unconscious need for self-punishment. Using imagery, we'll explore the personal meaning of these symptoms.

We're part of your team

This book is an extension of one of my pain centers, where the patients and staff function as a team. You are not the "patient," but the team member who is in pain or has a family member in pain. I am not the "doctor," some omniscient authority from afar, but the team member who teaches how to self-heal.

Combining state-of-the-art medicine, psychotherapeutic thinking and ways to help the individual search from within, **Pain Relief** enables you to take responsibility for your pain while it encourages the family to flourish and support the sufferer in healthy, constructive ways.

Perhaps your pain will not significantly subside after reading this book. You will nevertheless feel better about yourself and your situation. Rather than "learning to live with it," you will have learned to transcend pain, and even to appreciate its role in your life. That's my promise—and my guarantee!

Dr. Claude Amarnick

Introduction

> *Humpty Dumpty sat on a wall,*
> *Humpty Dumpty had a great fall.*
> *All the king's horses and all the king's men*
> *Couldn't put Humpty together again.*

Within days of establishing my rehabilitation medical practice in Queens, the truth behind the Humpty Dumpty nursery rhyme hit home. Millions of Americans in chronic pain were indeed Humpty Dumptys. Clearly, all the king's horses and all the king's men of modern medicine couldn't put Humpty together again. Nothing I had been taught in medical school or during my residencies in psychiatry and rehabilitation medicine had prepared me to help people in chronic pain.

The despairing sufferers who consulted me traveled from doctor to doctor, tried every remedy from aspirin and addictive analgesics to multiple surgeries. They had consulted psychiatrists, chiropractors, acupuncturists, homeopaths and physical therapists. The pain persisted. Why? These professionals had not assessed their patients' treatment history or organized a pain relief program that acknowledged the spiritual, psychological and social ramifications of pain. That, I discovered, was why these chronic pain sufferers continued to suffer. This was the beginning of my new career!

The impotency of American medicine

The statistics are shocking. Nearly one-third of all Americans are in constant pain—pain that accompanies back injuries and arthritis, as well as pain that has no apparent physical origin. For Americans, chronic pain is the most common cause of suffering and the main reason people visit a doctor or take medication.

In fact, chronic pain—pain that doesn't go away—confounds physicians far more than does acute pain. Unlike acute pain, which warns of disease or injury, chronic pain is usually unrelated to any apparent injury or illness. It cannot be visualized on X-ray or detected through physical examination or chemical tests. So doctors feel justified when they dismiss chronic pain as psychogenic (originating in the mind or emotions), especially when the standard remedies—bed rest, physical therapy, potent medications, nerve blocks and even surgery—all fail so miserably.

Chronic pain is one enormous public health problem. The International Association for the Study of Pain claims 40 million Americans are afflicted with arthritis, 70 million with back pain, and countless millions more with pain due to neck and joint injuries, sciatica and other long-term conditions.

The economics associated with chronic pain are also staggering. Chronic pain costs American business $70 billion annually in medical expenses, compensation claims and work days lost to illness and doctors' appointments. Chronic pain disables its victims for months at a stretch, and sometimes permanently. As a bowling ball knocks down pins, chronic pain wipes out the patient's physical, mental and emotional health, eroding family and work relationships and, frequently, finances.

Chronic pain patients quickly discover that our health system offers few answers. In fact, it magnifies their troubles, as chronic pain sufferers boomerang from one doctor to another, submitting to repetitive and mindless diagnostic evaluations. Many sufferers undergo unnecessary or even mutilating surgeries. Inevitably, they down a slew of prescriptions from different doctors. Powerful medications—Codeine, Percodan, Valium, Xanax, Nembutal—that carry the risk of drug addiction, poisoning and other dangerous side effects, are all routine. Still, these sufferers cannot find what causes their pain. Even worse, they cannot find relief.

A well-documented study from Seattle's University of Washington Medical Center says 86 percent of patients at the Washington Pain Clinic had no pathological diagnosis (no physical explanation for their pain). Yet forty percent underwent one or more surgical operations to relieve chronic pain. Eighty percent were taking more than one addictive pain medication. The pain persisted.

Preoccupied by patients with more tangible problems—like heart attacks and bleeding ulcers—general practitioners and internists have neither the time nor inclination to chart a patient's chronic pain or develop effective, perhaps innovative solutions for its control. This is particularly true when the pain is partly or entirely the expression of a psychic state like grief or fear, or when its sources are a mystery. Modern medicine has barely begun to recognize that chronic pain can be—and frequently is—psychogenic in origin.

Chronic pain patients are square pegs forced into round holes. Pain relief measures effectively used in emergencies for acute pain cannot be used indefinitely without addicting or even incapacitating the sufferer. But what are the alternatives? There are pain specialists, but only a few patients have the good fortune to be referred to them. When they are, it's by the more knowledgeable doctors, usually found in the handful of major cities that boast pain centers.

Sooner or later—after months or even years of fruitless search—a patient finally hears an exasperated doctor admit, "There's nothing I can do for you. It must be in your head. You'll just have to learn to live with it." What devastating news! Most chronic pain patients then feel betrayed and abused by the health care system they once considered their salvation. Then there are physicians who prescribe previously tried therapies, reinforcing the patient's feelings of hopelessness and depression. Some patients, particularly the highly anxious or severely depressed, contemplate suicide. A few act on it. The price of our impotency continues.

The more self-reliant sufferer discovers the growing number of self-help books on chronic pain—books that range from mainstream medical approaches to New Age healing. Most are incomplete or flawed. Many fraudulently guarantee freedom from pain or promise cures. False cures do the sufferer a great disservice. Still other self-help pain books are mechanistic, lack inspiration or are devoid of concrete treatments. The question continues: Why hasn't modern medicine come to grips with the overwhelming problem of chronic pain?

The answer lies in tradition

Pain historically has not been an important topic in medical research. Pain in the 1800s was itself considered a disease. Treat pain, medical thinking ran, and you treated disease. But as medical research discovered ailments that could be labeled, understood and treated, pain as a mere consequence assumed second place. Today, despite our many scientific advances and technology, no medical test or procedure to detect or measure pain has yet been found.

Chronic pain and the closely related subject of rehabilitation medicine still receive scant attention in medical school. Examine a standard hospital chart. You will still find no spot for a doctor or nurse to record whether a patient is experiencing chronic pain. But, more times than not, the pain is there.

Perhaps they knew more thousands of years ago, when Oriental holy men claimed they could consciously control their internal body functions. Western scientists and physicians consistently scoffed at these claims, preferring to treat the body as separate from the mind and spirit. But the mind-body-spirit approach re-educates the mind and body to overcome pain. It teaches you to examine what your pain means to you. It shows you how you can manage your pain so you can expect relief. It makes you responsible and able, not passive and helpless.

The pain management alternative

Medicine's failure to devise satisfactory alternative treatments impelled me to develop my own comprehensive pain management program. I became interested in rehabilitation medicine following my father's miraculous recovery from a ten-month coma. My first-hand observations of the mental, emotional and spiritual anguish that can accompany physical disability drove me to leave a thriving family practice to take residencies in both psychiatry and rehabilitation medicine. The first American physician in the United States board-certified in both specialties, I began my odyssey in the treatment of chronic pain.

For years meditation had helped me function at top capacity, even during difficult times. I found it a natural evolution to make meditation, elements of Eastern philosophy and Jungian thought key components of my pain management program. Here the individual transcends the perception of chronic pain and learns how to assume greater personal responsibility for managing his pain.

I believe that persistent pain signals deep internal conflict or disharmony. Pain was once considered a necessary component of the human condition, a "passion of the soul." My approach, on the other hand, emphasizes self-control over the fear of illness. According to Eastern philosophy, this control is the result of a lifelong effort to keep the mind calm and serene in the face of an emotional experience. It turns illness—one's deepest suffering—into an opportunity for growth.

When you explore your own spirituality, you will try to find and apply meaning to what happens to you each day. Human spirituality means finding a quiet, still, inner place where body, mind and spirit are in harmony. Your spiritual life enriches your daily life by giving it meaning and depth. Both Eastern and Western spiritual traditions teach that while your daily experience might seem chaotic and painful, you can find a connection and unifying principle at work in the universe. From that perspective, even your deepest suffering strengthens you.

On the other hand, untreated chronic pain wreaks spiritual havoc on a person, unsettling any sense of self. Depression, disability, financial stress, vocational difficulties and strained relationships are the consequences. The compounded distress loops into a vicious circle, heightening emotional and physical pain and creating a downward spiral. Pain patients relinquish more and more responsibility for their condition to their doctors as they become increasingly passive and dependent. Depression, with feelings of helplessness and hopelessness, is the unwelcome result of what I call the reverberating circuit.

Typically, those who suffer from depression due to chronic pain are inactive. They wait for someone to wave a magic wand to erase their pain. The thought of actively participating in their rehabilitation, of controlling their own pain, seldom crosses their minds. Because they use pain as an excuse, they shirk their responsibilities. Manipulation of others becomes their way of life. Soon they are isolated from others and from the activities they once enjoyed. The lack of any meaningful physical, social or recreational activities sinks them deeper into depression. The cycle spins. As pain increases in intensity, frequency or duration, depression follows the same path.

The opposite is also true: if the sufferer decreases his depression, the perception of pain will also decrease. Once he looks into his head as well as into his body, he realizes that his feelings of fear, helplessness, frustration, depression and anger—all learned from the pain—actually intensify and prolong that pain.

Get up, get moving

That's why I urge you to become active. Try specific exercises. Increase your activity level by abandoning the television set for something more physical, whether it's a walk around the block, window shopping or a bicycle ride. Learn how to get on your feet by choosing an activity you can physically handle and enjoy.

I will teach you that the more you worry about depression, the worse it becomes. Specific exercises in this book will show you how not to fall into the trap of focusing on your depression. To actively remove depression from your life is your crucial first step. Case histories, combined with new research, substantiate my steps for controlling your chronic pain.

In the pages to come, you will learn how to:

•Control pain—not be controlled by it

•Master the pain/depression/insomnia cycle by intelligently combining medication, deceleration and exercise

•Turn positive thinking and behavior patterns into a new physical self

•Tap your inner resources through creative visualization and meditation

By learning what pain is and how the pain cycle develops, you will discover how it operates in your particular situation and how the events of your daily life, working through your emotions, affect you physically.

This book introduces issues vital to your understanding and treatment of chronic pain. You will learn that your pain is not a disease or the effect of a disease, but a sensory experience. This means it can be altered by the way you interpret it. Unmanageable chronic pain is an assault on your autonomy and competence. This book offers methods to maximize your feelings of autonomy and competence.

My guarantee

There is no cure for chronic pain. Recovering from chronic pain is a gradual healing process. Apart from its psychological and spiritual origins, there is almost always a physiological reason that causes chronic pain to persist or recur. I will not promise that this book will make your pain disappear, but I do guarantee that by following my innovative program you too can learn to control your pain rather than let it control you. You will lose the hapless sense that pain has taken over your personality and runs your life. Consulting your inner guide is really a matter of uncovering feelings you may not be fully aware of and clarifying what you really need or want.

In Eastern medicine and philosophy, patients are encouraged to accept rather than fight the pain experience. This practice helps the patient transform pain by facing it and making peace with it.

In addition to physical pain, individuals with chronic pain are also in spiritual pain. Drugs and multiple surgeries do not relieve this inner anguish. In this book you will learn alternatives to medication and alcohol. When you no longer depend upon these substances, you are no longer dependent on pain.

This book reflects my conviction that the special problem and constitutional makeup of chronic pain patients require equal doses of concrete solutions and their own very real accomplishments. As the pages that follow will show, there are unlimited possibilities to lead a full, productive life, despite your pain.

*Nothing succeeds like success: You will find, one day,
that you have rediscovered hope!*

Taking Charge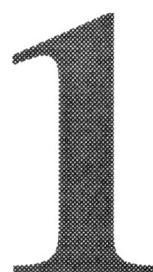

The average doctor sees 40-50 patients in a five-hour day. Understandably he has neither the time nor interest to assume total responsibility for his patients' health. As a result, no one becomes pain manager for the chronic pain patient, a sufferer who drifts from one fruitless doctor's appointment to another. The medical system's treatment of chronic pain creates a vicious catch-22 for all involved. Meanwhile, prescriptions for bed rest, physical therapy, potent medications, nerve blocks and surgery make patients passively dependent on their doctors.

Health care practitioners are now awakening to chronic pain as a medical entity. Some day the importance of pain management will be reflected in professional training and new approaches to pain treatment. But today there remains a vast gap between patients' beliefs in their physicians' omnipotence and the reality: Doctors know very little about chronic pain.

Even doctors admit that less than 15 percent of all illness is treatable scientifically, and that the medical community cannot help seven out of ten patients. But most physicians have a difficult time accepting that. It contradicts their medical training and role expectations. Almost in cookbook fashion, physicians are trained to pinpoint illness and apply the proper prescription—whether it be drugs or therapy—as though following a foolproof cake recipe. They expect an immediate cure. When cookbook medicine fails, they can deal with their frustration in one of two ways: blame the patient or blame themselves. Since it is human nature to fault others, the patient becomes a scapegoat.

Chronic pain can throw even the veteran physician into ambivalence. It should be the opportunity for the doctor to travel uncharted waters of holistic medicine, to incorporate the tenets of Eastern philosophy. But instead of recognizing the wholeness of the individual and the dynamic interworkings of body with mind, most physicians attribute illnesses they cannot define as "all in the patient's head." Thus, the doctor preserves his omnipotence and infallibility.

Perhaps most damaging to the individual is that since the physician has learned to rely on drugs as a cookbook ingredient, he need not send the patient away untreated. He prescribes happiness in the form of tranquilizing capsules, or doles out relief in sleeping pills or painkillers.

The self is forgotten

The doctor still has not made the patient well. He has not even considered the possibility that the individual's chronic pain might arise from a malfunction between mind, body and spirit. The self is the forgotten ingredient in the recipe. Cookbook medicine—following a designated formula—is easier than a search for the control of chronic pain. For this there is no proven recipe.

When physicians say pain is "in your head," they are right. Chronic pain is in your mind as much as in the injured tissue. Holistic medicine accepts that "in your head" is a perfectly respectable place for pain. Therefore, if you want to control your chronic pain, it's wise to look into the depths of your mind and soul as well as into your physical being. It's important to examine your perception of pain, to find out the extent to which fear, helplessness, frustration, depression and anger—learned from pain—are intensifying and prolonging it.

Because pain cannot now be directly measured, individuals in chronic pain frequently ask if their pain is "real." Most physicians distinguish between real and imaginary pain. They have established a hierarchy that puts body over mind, thus conditioning how society thinks about health and disease.

Pain has a dual problem: It is immeasurable, and it is made up of physical as well as perceptual and psychological aspects. It is thus poorly understood as an integrated entity. But one thing is clear: separating mind from body can never give us the answer to chronic pain.

Hopefully one day physicians will replace anxiety with confidence, and hopelessness with hope. These physicians will empathize with, listen to and help the sufferer unburden his feelings of guilt, worthlessness, fear and anger. The medical community will then have truly embraced the concept of chronic pain management.

Identifying your emotional component and understanding that you must become an active participant in your recovery is the first step in stopping the reverberating circuit. Start a simple notebook as you go through this book. Use it to answer questions as they arise and to record your thoughts and the degree of your pain. Also use it for the exercises I suggest throughout the book.

To create your chronic pain control program, you must recognize that the critical measure of responsibility for the control of your pain rests on your shoulders. Look first at your social problems. What social interactions trouble you? How does your chronic pain cause, increase and/or interfere with these problems? Be honest about your problems and be committed to treating every aspect of your health. Avoid the lure of easy cures. You will soon gain mastery over your pain.

Discovering the factors that contribute to your chronic pain takes strict discipline. It means genuinely caring about your health—a responsibility you must not take lightly.

Exercise: Ask yourself these questions:

1. What is happening inside my mind at this moment?

2. Where is my awareness at this moment?

3. How present am I when I am engaged in my everyday activities?

4. How will I transcend my perception of pain?

Awareness is training the mind and the body to be present in the now. You will do exactly that throughout this book.

Yes, it takes courage, self-confidence and trust to understand and accept your feelings and inner thoughts. But it is necessary. As you accept your pain not as punishment but as a call for deeper awareness, you will find a greater harmony in your life.

Understanding chronic pain as a warning flag—a helpful signal—allows you to look at your situation differently and find an honest way to cope with it.

Occasionally you may deny or suppress your feelings about your chronic pain. Or you may choose a non-confrontational path to hide from it. Instead, work toward self-awareness. The world of feelings can be a fertile arena for self-discovery, inner transformation and healing.

Exercise: Ask yourself these four questions. Write your answers in your notebook. Please don't ignore this exercise. Give each question your full consideration. If you don't know, write "I don't know."

1. How do you usually deal with your feelings?

2. What feelings call for expression or attention?

3. What fears have kept you from acknowledging those feelings?

4. Do you have the strength to follow your heart if it guides you to a different path?

Inner peace is attainable. It comes from the awareness that our satisfaction in living does not result from what happens to us, but from our thoughts. We make of life what we want. Your pain management program is not based on overt behavior; it is based on the principle that your attitude determines your perceptions and sensations.

Look inward

Coping with chronic pain must come from within. Individuals with chronic pain often believe they are powerless, unloved and lost. Belief is a very powerful force. Belief in the power of your inner soul and spirit is crucial. It is the core of your self-esteem. If you find that you do not believe or when you feel that all is wasted and unused, look inward for your innate skills, talents, courage and strength.

The power of positive emotions has enormous potential to heal. You have the strength and opportunity to become what you want to be. It is time to become yourself. Nurture yourself physically, emotionally and spiritually. You hold this power.

My patients frequently begrudge taking any time for a quiet introspection on their lives. I call this "resisting a rest." But tranquility is the inner lining of every activity in your life. Do what brings you happiness. This is where you find your inner peace. Everyone has a personal path that he or she must follow. Only when you find the courage to follow your course will you find inner peace and contentment.

Exercise:

1. Think about the times in your life when you "resisted a rest."

2. List these times. Highlight specific times when you felt particularly rushed and harried.

3. Recount the opportunities that could create space for a more joyful life. Include specific activities that you do for your own sheer enjoyment and/or interest.

Exercise: Ask yourself these seven important questions.

1. What are you doing now that you don't completely believe in?

2. How could this be contributing to your chronic pain?

3. What activities would you prefer doing?

4. How might these relieve your chronic pain?

5. When you do or say something that you do not believe in, do you feel increased stress and pain?

6. Do you feel you are merely existing, rather than living a life that expresses your true feelings, wants and desires?

7. Do you feel your chronic pain is worse when you have such feelings?

Barbara

A serious motor vehicle accident caused Barbara acute neck pain and some mid-back muscle spasticity and discomfort. The pain deteriorated into an agonizing chronic situation, and Barbara lost a considerable amount of range of motion in her neck. The pain radiated from her neck into her shoulders and eventually into her arms. She underwent extensive diagnostic tests from various physicians and was prescribed various addictive pain-killers.

Soon Barbara's days consisted entirely of journeying from one physician to another, without coordination or "triage" among them. In fact, no one physician treating her knew what medications the others were prescribing. Barbara was exhausted from her role of helpless patient. She wouldn't undertake active physical therapy, because she was increasingly convinced that she had become an invalid. She regressed until she became totally dependent on the health care system.

Four years after her motor vehicle accident, Barbara came to our multi-disciplinary pain center. I knew immediately that Barbara needed an array of activities other than that of "waiting room occupant." Barbara soon reduced the intensity of her chronic pain by her own assertive coping efforts. She learned substitution: Avoiding accentuating pain by replacing emotional distress with calm. Barbara distracted herself from pain by visualizing only the most pleasant and peaceful scenes. For example, she would say to herself:

"I see a meadow brushing up against a clear blue sky. The sun is bright, yielding strong rays of penetrating warmth. The light makes the tall grass glisten. A soft breeze lifts the blades harmoniously, like the waves on a lake rippled by a canoe.

"I lie down in the womb of the meadow, protected by the tall grass. The sun's warmth penetrates my body. First, it gently pierces my skin, and finally it penetrates deep into my organs. My entire body, from its central core out, feels incredibly warm, happy, relaxed. I hear birds and a single cricket. I stay here forever; peaceful eternity at last. I am at one with my surroundings." In moments, Barbara was relaxed, her pain forgotten.

In order to imagine her pain, Barbara would say, "The pain is like rats gnawing at my neck and mid-back." Or "like a woodpecker drilling at the skin in my neck." Or "like red-hot flashes of metal with jagged points touching and piercing my back."

Barbara deftly transformed her images of pain. The gnawing rat faded away. Her imagination slowly transformed pain by changing her perception of pain. Finally, relaxation and relief replaced overwhelming anxiety.

Barbara exercised this technique at home, several times each day. It was essential that she adhere to a regular schedule, developed from the daily ups and downs of her pain as recorded in her notebook. Whenever she anticipated pain, she learned to block it with the substitution technique. Replacing her anxiety with calm, she gave her mind, spirit and body an important message.

Try the substitution technique. Follow Barbara's steps. You might place yourself in a cornfield and imagine hearing the crack of dry corn stalks. Whatever you visualize, you goal is to develop a feel for the process.

Debra

Debra, an attractive 35-year-old bank executive, shows how even intelligent, successful individuals become alarmingly passive with their medical practitioners. Debra needed self-man agement training to assume greater responsibility for managing her health. Instead, like most individuals with chronic pain, Debra delegated this to a physician or therapist. And, quite possibly like yourself, she became the helpless victim.

Debra had seen several physicians for her head, jaw and neck pain over two and a half years. She tried many therapies and medications before she walked into my chronic pain multi-disciplinary center. She had lost faith in herself and in her ability to control her life.

When I met Debra she was totally demoralized by her reduced physical activity, listlessness and diminished social life. She no longer wanted to socialize, which fed her depression. Her life got out of control as Debra lost all incentive, couldn't think straight, couldn't cope. In a deep rut, Debra felt helpless.

As University of Pennsylvania psychology professor Dr. Martin Seligman says, the more helpless people feel when placed in situations beyond their control, the more helpless they become. He calls this "learned helplessness." Understand this and you understand that, to adapt to pain, you must believe in your ability to control it. I will reiterate throughout this book how important it is for you to shed the stigma of learned helplessness. I will teach you every technique I know to rid yourself of these conditioned responses to events that trigger your chronic pain.

When you cannot control a stressful situation, you develop more anxiety, stress, tension and pain. Constant tension produces harmful physiological effects, including more chronic pain. Tension at work, for example, may make it difficult to concentrate. It may impair your judgment so you make incorrect decisions. Tension consumes energy and can lead to extreme fatigue at day's end, producing insomnia and physical illness such as chronic pain. But tension does even more damage. Because you cannot control it, you feel helpless and think less of yourself. Your self-esteem spirals downward.

Turn off the tension

To ease tension, learn how to relax. Begin by telling yourself, when necessary, "Relax." Then do it. This active approach helps you overcome the tension. The key? Know your tensions and switch them off. Through relaxation exercises you command life's stresses. With self-control—that is, control over the stimulus— you relieve pain. The stimuli that trigger your chronic pain are small events, but they can trigger a big reaction.

Stress is important with chronic pain sufferers, because stress has physical repercussions. Need proof? Look at your muscle tension or how you breathe. One sign of stress is heightened muscle tension, which directly effects chronic pain. Correct these abnormalities and you reduce your chronic pain. Yes, the physical symptoms of stress are unpleasant, alarming and, more importantly, exhausting. When your body undergoes prolonged stress, you reduce your ability to cope with life or pain.

Reducing stress enables you to increase your coping skills. Three simple steps to manage stressful events:

1. Identify your stress triggers.

2. Write them down.

3. Learn to recognize when stress affects you.

To reduce the physical symptoms of stress you must learn how to relax using progressive muscle relaxation, breathing control and mind-calming techniques. View a stressful situation as a cue to relax. Use the relaxation exercises in this book several times a day. Positive inner dialogues help manage your stress triggers. Why let minor daily hassles make you feel uptight and suffer the repercussions of stress?

Your symptoms are real

Make no mistake: your symptoms are very real. Physical effects like rapid breathing and increased muscle tension both increase your pain and decrease your ability to cope with it. Overbreathing produces physical symptoms due to a reduced level of carbon dioxide in the body. It also produces stress, which leads to heightened muscle tension and an increase in your chronic pain. So the pain triggers stress, and you're quickly on the reverberating circuit.

Unfortunately, stress is a fact of life. Everyone feels stressed occasionally. When you feel stressed, recognize it and do not pretend that all is well. Instead, use the techniques in the book to take action.

Depression is common in individuals with chronic pain, a result of prolonged pain, frustration and anger. There are many signs of depression.

Exercise: Is depression a key factor in your chronic pain? Answer eight questions:

1. Do you feel hopeless? Does life look bleak or appear to be a long dark tunnel?

2. Do you feel powerless? Do your efforts seem to be in vain and inadequate to change your life?

3. Do you feel worthless or that your life is without merit or value?

4. Do you have trouble either falling or staying asleep? Do you have disturbing dreams or a sense of dread?

5. Do you eat poorly?

6. Do you have a sexual disorder—either an inability to perform or a lack of desire?

7. Do you feel confused, with mental haziness or an inability to concentrate on daily matters?

8. Do you often feel sad, bleak or tearful? Does your life seem bland? Have you lost interest in most activities? Do you wish you weren't alive? Do you feel suicidal? Is there a heaviness or pall, or an isolation and withdrawal, that it is overwhelming?

Pain magnifies depression, and depression magnifies pain. If you answered yes to two or more of the above questions, the likelihood is significant that you do or will experience depression along with chronic pain.

The single most important thing you can do to avoid or minimize depression's debilitating effect is to seek companionship and meaningful social interaction. Those with chronic pain are natural victims of isolation, and frequently spend much of their non-working hours at home. Isolation at first is physical, but rapidly becomes mental. Individuals who are alone soon feel ashamed, embarrassed, confused. They lose perspective and feel helpless and misunderstood. They then retreat to the comfort of bed, both to avoid pain and to soothe their minds. It's tempting to hide. More depression makes it easier to yield to this temptation and increase isolation.

Demand success

Depression. Helplessness. Hopelessness. They each indicate a lack of confidence in your own ability. It's common for confidence to erode quickly with chronic pain. Anticipating hurt imparts an anxiety that prevents action. By performing the exercises I outline, you can get a firm grip on your expectations, anticipate your reactions and thereby control your chronic pain.

Expectation is what you imagine the consequence of your actions to be. Expect favorable outcomes and you will take risks to achieve them. Expect poor outcomes and you will hold back. Chronic pain sufferers usually hold back; they rarely expect success. Instead, they play a waiting game.

When you lack the tools to control chronic pain, your confidence drops, anxiety increases and the downward spiral starts. Because pain is perceived to be beyond your control, you become angry, producing muscle spasm. Pain increases, grinding down endurance, eroding confidence and producing further expectations of failure. You must stop this spiral!

To control your body and your chronic pain you must take charge and make choices. Experience failure and you will feel no control over your pain. Instead, passivity and powerlessness control your attitude. Your aim is simple: Develop a broad repertoire of coping strategies. Each will help you regain and retain mastery over your environment and pain.

Exercise: To regain control and mastery over your environment, list in your notebook the "up" things you can and like to do. When depression starts, go through the items on the list. Create a daily checklist. Use the above substitution technique to replace depressing thoughts with ideas that make you happy.

Your journal should be specific and realistic about your goals. You may never be completely pain-free, but you can loosen pain's grip as positive aspects of your life push aside the negative. Too little positive reinforcement in your life may be because you have created a lifestyle with too few opportunities for positive reinforcement. You may have created a situation where good things cannot happen. Instead, you have chosen to center your life around negative reinforcements. Switch gears! Try positive reinforcements to keep unpleasant things from happening, or bad things from becoming worse.

So, the best way to combat depression is through positive reinforcement. Seek new sources of pleasure—things that will provide you with a positive view of the world around you. Choose activities that can most satisfy you. Enhance and cherish your positive feelings.

One characteristic of depression is the inability to act. To effectively manage your depression you must:

1. Carefully analyze your daily activities.

2. Change your lifestyle to get involved and interact with people. Increasing mobility is important in managing chronic pain. More activity not only increases your self-confidence, but also affects your mood, thanks to the body's endorphins.

3. Reward yourself when you actively engage in activities or become involved with others.

4. Recognize negative thoughts and feelings and convert them to positive ones. Convince yourself that your thoughts and feelings are within your conscious control. Challenge unpleasant thoughts and emotions. Then substitute them

with positive ones. Don't spend energy on being upset. Look at the situation differently. Step back, analyze and focus your energy into thinking and feeling positively.

Exercise: Try this exercise if you feel gloomy. It's a lesson in seeking positive reinforcement through fantasy and imagery.

1. Imagine the activities that would give you pleasure. Systematically consider hobbies, entertainment, sports, sex, social interactions, travel and other categories.

2. List your choices in your notebook.

3. Do this exercise daily until you can move from the imagination stage to the willingness stage to the doing stage. Your immediate goal is to relieve your depression sufficiently so that you can live life instead of imagining life. Your long-term goal is to fight depression with activity rather than with fantasy.

4. Make it a habit to do more things you enjoy. In fact, make it a daily ritual.

Chronic pain sufferers often have such strong negative feelings that they cannot be assertive. Feelings of anger, worry, frustration, guilt, jealousy, depression and inadequacy are, of course, negative and unproductive. They make it difficult for you to behave as you want. So instead of acting out good feelings, you sabotage yourself with chronic pain.

But you can counteract negativity with imagery. Indeed, imagery as a tool for assertiveness is an idea whose time has come. Imagery can reduce your fears and achieve what you want. Combine imagery with assertiveness and you can manage your pain. You heal. Try it: Imagine a something pleasant, perhaps lying on a beach, sitting in a pleasant garden, relaxing in a bath.

Focus on the feelings in your chest as you slowly and steadily inhale and exhale.

You must learn how to relax using progressive muscle relaxation and techniques to control breathing and calm the mind. Tackling stress takes time, but it is time well spent. You learn to cope and may be able to reduce the chronic pain caused by muscular tension.

To express to others what you think and feel, you must be assertive. Assertiveness gives you more confidence and control. You then feel less helpless to change what causes your pain. Use these methods and you are well armed to change how you think and move on to a life no longer dominated by chronic pain. Assertiveness is discussed in detail in the next chapter.

There is a direct link between your feelings and your thinking, which reconnects to your feelings. ("I hurt, therefore I am unable, therefore I am a victim, therefore I hurt.") Your feelings do not arise from nowhere. They are the result of an external situation and your thoughts.

This is the reverberating circuit I continuously mention. The reverberating circuit holds the key to pain management. Cut this reverberating circuit, and you can control your chronic pain—and heal. Your feelings are not controlled by events or by others. You control them. You alone have this great opportunity to gain more control of your feelings—not to stifle them, or give them free rein, but to change them in any way you wish, and express them openly and honestly. When you do, you bring your feelings within your control and "own" them.

When bad feelings pay dividends

Many people who have unproductive feelings may actually experience secondary gains—that is, rewards that follow their feelings. They then repeat these feelings, dropping those that do not lead to a gain. Over time these feelings become habit, part of their "feelings repertoire," even when these feelings sabotage the individual.

The "rewarded feelings" I speak about are difficult to identify, but those who feel helpless, inadequate, rejected, miserable and angry often are comfortable harboring such feelings. There is familiarity in the self-fulfilling effects of what you believe about yourself. ("This is who I am: I hurt, therefore I am unable, therefore I am a victim, therefore I hurt.")

These feelings can be consciously controlled, but it's not easy, particularly as it relates to chronic pain. Feelings that become habit are so deeply rooted that you do not realize you actually chose them.

As a chronic pain sufferer, you must unlearn an entire abnormal lifestyle that pain has taught you. Your pain won't stop, but you won't let it control you as it recedes in importance. Although pain has dominated your existence, you must now believe you can escape pain and, like Humpty Dumpty, put your life back together again. You must have the courage of your convictions to regain your self-esteem and independence. Trust your judgment. That's how you control chronic pain. But nothing succeeds like success: You will find, one day, that you have rediscovered hope!

The specific exercises in this book will reinforce that hope. If you relax, your perception of pain becomes altered. You can learn how to meditate, use imagery, relax, breathe deeply and practice creative visualization, and you can do it without having to enter a residential treatment center. When motivated, you can become your own best doctor.

Also recognize that you are wasting your anger. It only makes your life worse. Turn that anger around and it can fuel your determination to conquer pain and regain control of your life. You achieve this by embracing a fundamental self-help premise: The spirit, the mind and the body must all be healthy in unison to find inner peace and contentment. To achieve deep physical relaxation, you must achieve mental relaxation. Both need practice.

You also can no longer resist holistic medicine. You may know intellectually that good health depends on being well in mind as well as in body, but you may also dismiss meditation, relaxation and self-examination as too mystical, and consequently dismiss holistic medicine without even understanding it.

Holistic medicine believes you are responsible for your own health. Not only can you control your behavior, but you can learn to keep fundamental body processes—like pulse rate, temperature, blood pressure and digestion—in good order. Chronic pain is one such body process you can learn to control.

Treating physical symptoms is not enough. This book also teaches you how to combine physical, mental, emotional and spiritual disciplines into a personalized treatment. Your pain management program will support you and your family in making the life changes that healing pain requires.

Letting go is enormously liberating.
When you open up, others will start opening up to you.

Setting Goals, Being Assertive

2

Assertiveness training can explicate you from learned helplessness. The dictionary defines assertion as "an affirmation, a declaration, or a positive statement; insistence upon a right." Assertion means expressing your needs, wants, opinions, feelings and beliefs in direct, honest and appropriate ways.

Do you have trouble saying what you mean and expressing your needs? Are you fearful of rejection? By practicing assertiveness techniques you learn to express displeasure and ask for what you want. As you do this, you'll find anxiety and anger melting away. At the same time, you'll discover that being direct has positive effect on other modes of behavior.

Learning to become assertive is one of the most important exercises in this book. When you are assertive, you are in touch with your feelings and you tap into your subconscious. This enables you to move on. You give yourself permission to "own" your feelings. You become more confident in handling life's situations, including your chronic pain. And that, after all, is what this book is all about: controlling the perception and sensation of chronic pain.

Doing exercises to become more assertive helps you deal with a real problem; it also teaches you how to manage and control your own health situation. The goal is to discuss what you consider unpleasant topics, instead of bottling them up for fear of offending or losing love. This may be in violation of the childhood code of behavior that you still follow even though it is counterproductive for you.

Not being assertive has negative effects for you, including a loss of self-esteem. There is a direct relationship between assertiveness and self-esteem. Self-esteem is the value you perceive about yourself. When you are unable to take initiatives or face up to difficult situations, you become angry or frustrated with yourself, feel hurt, or drop into sustained self-pity. These feelings are directed inward, and lead to increased stress and internal tensions. The result is exacerbation of your chronic pain.

After a few practice sessions, you will find that you are quite able to say and feel what you wish. When you are direct with people—as long as you are considerate and fair—you create trust, friendship and a comfortable, easy atmosphere. You have replaced what you thought would create hostility with effective communication and interchange. This interplay teaches you important lessons about being in control of your life.

Letting go is liberating

Being assertive means finding a more constructive way of expressing yourself. Letting go is enormously liberating. When you open up, others will start opening up to you. The work on attitudes and feelings, on how you see yourself and how you get along with those around you, is all done to achieve the program's single-minded goal: teaching you to take responsibility.

The process of becoming assertive is comparable to learning a foreign language. At first you master words, phrases, ground rules. Mastering the language of assertion requires knowing what assertive behavior is; practicing its principles, rules and regulations; and, most importantly, applying it daily in your life. Many individuals have trouble with assertiveness because they don't understand what it is, avoid assertive situations, or never learned the behavior.

The assertive exercises you learn here center on how to set your own goals and sub-goals. These exercises help overcome any communication difficulties you might have that prevent you from expressing your needs.

Your first step is developing a goal system. This means creating an action plan for yourself. Without goals, you lack a sense of purpose and motivation. Goals reinforce self-esteem: achievement of goals strengthens your desire to achieve other goals. As a result, you move through life with a higher sense of self-worth.

You need to set both short-term and long-term goals. Set up a series of sub (short-term) goals. If you select a distant goal without sub-goals, you fail to see progress or develop a sense of accomplishment, and you become discouraged. Goals provide you with a more positive identity.

Exercise: Think of an idealized image of yourself, the kind of individual you would like to become. Close your eyes and imagine that idealized self. Smell that idealized self, see him, hear his voice, feel the texture of his skin. Become totally consumed with all the traits and qualities you would like to possess.

Open your eyes and write in your notebook a description of the kind of person you want to be. Be concrete. List your ideal characteristics in order of importance to you. Keep writing until you have eight to ten qualities. Read over your list several times, until you have it clearly memorized. Close your eyes once again. Feel that idealized self. Remember each and every trait you wrote down. Next, list in your notebook how you can become that idealized self. Go through the list. If there is a big discrepancy between you now and you as you'd like to be, what can you do to develop those desired traits?

We concentrate on behavior, beliefs, thoughts and feelings because they can be changed. It is not easy, but it can be done. With practice, you change your behavior. After awhile your new behavior becomes natural, and you realize that your feelings and beliefs have also changed. By approaching this in small steps, listing sub-goals for yourself to follow, change will occur.

Know your limitations

Make your goals realizations of your essential abilities. Start slowly, by subdividing seemingly massive goals. By breaking them into sub-goals, you make it easier to succeed one step at a time.

Exercise: This exercise considers impersonal situations; then work, job or business situations; and lastly, the most complicated: social interactions. Look for opportunities to interact with family members, friends, acquaintances and neighbors. Count the number of times you express your feelings in those interactions in one week. In the same way, search out opportunities to express displeasure or annoyance, if indeed these people do something that annoys or displeases you.

In social interactions you must communicate with another person what you are feeling at the moment in a direct, honest and appropriate way. By doing this, you become a more alive individual, more sensitive to and aware of your own feelings and more open to the feelings of others. Learning to become assertive entails changing behavior by dealing with what is already there. What's important is the content of one's communication. Consider the feelings that you are trying to express. Concentrate on stating exactly what you think.

When you are not assertive, you are not focused on the things you consider important and the goals you wish to obtain. You become so burdened doing the things you don't want to do that you have neither time or energy for the things that are most important to you. You are merely existing, performing tasks that others wish you to do. You feel exploited; resentments build up and you begin to manifest all of this in unhealthy ways, including developing chronic pain.

You are learning how to handle situations differently than you have in the past. This means behaving assertively, as opposed to meekly or aggressively. But first, understand your rights. If you do not know what your rights are, you will find it difficult to judge whether other people are violating these rights. Knowing your rights makes it possible to express yourself in a free and assertive manner. Your rights include:

•having your own opinions, views and ideas

•getting a fair hearing for these opinions, views and ideas

•having needs and wants that may be different from others'

•expressing those needs assertively

•being your own self

Your filter on the world

Your beliefs about yourself directly affect your actions and behavior. They are strongly linked to your feelings and influence the way you interpret the results of your actions. They are your filter on the world; you seek out things that reinforce your beliefs and ignore or explain away things that do not fit your beliefs.

Exercise: Holding true to your beliefs increases your chances to learn new behavior. This exercise involves using assertive statements in your everyday actions. Write the following statements in your notebook:

1. I am responsible for what happens to me.

2. I am in control, I can choose how to behave.

3. I can change.

4. I can initiate actions to achieve results.

5. I can learn from feedback.

6. I believe assertiveness works.

Writing these statements down forces you to consider their truth. This is a chance to learn new guidelines for your behavior. Thus, being clear on and "owning" your rights provides a basis for assertive behavior.

You become assertive by practicing and using assertiveness tools in a step-by-step fashion. Start with short interactions with fairly straightforward outcomes. Warning: It isn't easy! Often, individuals with chronic pain are unable to state their wants and desires because they have not learned how to ask for what they want. The following situations provide hints for behaving assertively.

1. Make a request in a straightforward, open way. Be direct. Keep it short; long-winded explanations get confusing and increase the chances that you will start justifying yourself.

2. Give a reason for your request if you think it will help.

3. Don't take a refusal personally, even when the request is of a personal nature. Respect the other person's right to say no.

4. Equally important, learn how to say no to others' requests. As with making requests, any difficulties you may have in saying "No" stem from the beliefs you hold. Hints for refusing requests assertively:

   A. Keep the reply short but not abrupt.

   B. Try phrases like "I prefer not to ...", "I'd rather not ..," "No, I don't want to ...," or "I'm not happy to ..."

   C. Give an honest reason for refusing. Do not invent an excuse.

Assertive behavior involves agreeing and disagreeing without leading to conflict. This is important, because conflict instills tension, stress and anxiety. Any of these factors can lead to an exacerbation of your chronic pain.

When you learn to stand up for your point of view, your need to sabotage yourself and others is greatly diminished. Thus, the likelihood of having an exacerbation of chronic pain greatly decreases. Learn how to state your opinion, whether it is similar or different from others.

If you never reveal your true self, you can never be comfortable with others. Learning to become assertive teaches you how important the spontaneous expression of feelings is. After all, feelings are not isolated emotions; they are incorporated and integrated into the threads that make up each one of us. Ideally, becoming assertive blends your thoughts, actions and feelings into a unified individual. This is all part of the mind-body-spirit approach to healthy integration.

Role-playing

Are you able to say no when you want? In role-playing, you rehearse how to say "No" in a direct, efficient and effective manner. Imagine an unpleasant situation you might find yourself in, and develop responses that change and diffuse that situation. You do this by response rehearsal. Perhaps you've never clearly thought out how you wish to respond. Perhaps, because you have never learned to use an assertive response, you act unassertively. By practicing them over and over, you become comfortable with your responses; they are so natural that they become a part of you. Role-playing simulates reality in a protected environment. Eventually you can take what you learn and put it to use in real life.

Exercise: This exercise teaches you how to say "No." Instead of building up resentments that manifest themselves as chronic pain, you develop your own style of stating negative responses.

Define those areas in your life where you have trouble saying "No," role-play those situations and rate your progress. Conjuring up ways to change your behavior is not the hard part; it's rating yourself that tends to cause the most inner discomfort!

Every morning ask yourself, "What are my priorities for today?" This will be a map for your day. You need to have a vision, a purpose and a goal to take you through this exercise. Then you need to take action. Have the discipline to make your priorities a part of your day. After all, to manage and control requires acknowledging the value of your goals. For a week, set aside time each day to contemplate what is important for you in resolving your pain. Writing in your journal establishes priorities and begins to map out a path to accomplishing them.

Actually performing the tasks you've set for yourself takes time, work, effort, discipline and a willingness to change. Ask yourself the most fundamental of questions: What are my deepest purposes? How can I help and what can I contribute?

Exercise: To prioritize your life and handle your chronic pain, ask yourself these questions. Again, record your feelings in your notebook.

1. Do I confront the real issues behind my chronic pain?

2. Have I thought of solutions that can resolve my chronic pain?

3. Have I found avenues to communicate feelings other than suffering from my chronic pain?

4. Have I behaved differently, and have I requested that others react toward me in new, constructive ways?

5. How am I going to focus my energy so that I am best able to control and manage my chronic pain?

6. How can I measure my success? (There must be no pretending or bluffing with this one. You need to be able to measure your success in some way.)

7. Who in my life is depending on me? Can I rely on myself to follow my commitments? Since we are all interconnected, there must be a thread of commitment and caring linking human beings. Ask yourself how a successful resolution of your chronic pain can help you deal with these broader human interests.

8. What am I forgetting or ignoring? What areas in life do I need to sharpen up on? By continuously expressing my chronic pain, what is cloudy, or foggy, or being covered up? You must be very clear that you, alone, make things happen in your life. Don't be vague. Once you stop ignoring these areas, you'll spring forward quite swiftly.

Do these exercises with a passion. It is from passion and the investment of all of your energies that you succeed. You can heal. If you follow the exercises in this chapter on how to be assertive, your level of self-esteem will be greatly enhanced. From this new level, your ability to manage and control your chronic pain increases, as does the healing process.

You can feel like a healthy person,
even if your pain persists!

Jim's Story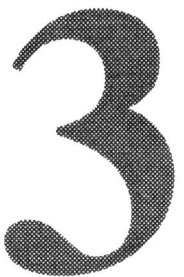

You know pain management demands your active involvement. My program lessens your dependency on drugs and doctors. As Jim's story illustrates, nothing but misery comes from taking drugs, lying in bed, hoping your pain subsides. Repeated failures are plentiful, as patient and physician blame the other.

Jim

Jim, a 45-year-old accountant, endured increasingly sharp lower back pain for 21 years. He needed more from me than a prescription or positive bedside manner. Jim couldn't precisely remember when his back started to hurt, but he believed it was when he was in his early twenties, fresh out of school, newly married and holding down a promising new job.

"I think it happened just as everything was beginning to go right for the first time," Jim recalled wistfully.

Jim's case history went full circle, starting with years of unsuccessful treatment with traditional medicine. After pursuing my comprehensive pain management program, he repaired his battered self-image, reunited with his family and greatly lessened his pain. Our collaboration was crucial to his recovery. You, too, should find a doctor who will work with you as part of a multidisciplinary team. You'll feel much better than if you blindly do as a doctor recommends or force a doctor to prescribe drugs or perform unnecessary surgery.

When Jim first experienced pain, he consulted his family doctor, a general practitioner, who referred him to an internist. The internist prescribed tranquilizers, muscle relaxants, ice packs and strict bed rest. The pain persisted. Jim's second internist, highly recommended by a co-worker, prescribed a different drug, maintained that moist heat, hot baths and heat pads were better than cold treatments, and urged Jim to exercise regularly.

Confused by his two internists' contradictory advice, and continuing to feel pain, Jim consulted still more experts. For years he faithfully followed their advice. None brought more than temporary relief. An orthopedic surgeon suggested traction and, if that failed, disc surgery. A chiropractor told him surgery was a mistake—chiropractic adjustments five times a week were the answer. A fellow sufferer recommended a health spa that specialized in back rehabilitation. An anesthesiologist offered to numb Jim's pain temporarily with a nerve block. Finally, after much pressure from family and friends, Jim saw a psychiatrist. After he told the psychiatrist, "I wish my boss would get off my back" and that having three college-bound children made him feel like "I have the weight of the world on my shoulders," she deduced that Jim's pain was a symptom of emotional disturbance and recommended intensive therapy.

But after years of failed treatment, Jim's life began to fall apart. Muscle spasm severely limited his movements. He called in sick so frequently that he feared losing his job. His office mates grumbled because they had to handle his load and had tired of his endless war stories of pain and doctors. Jim, resenting their lack of sympathy, became irritable with them. His pain prevented him from thinking clearly about office assignments and responsibilities.

Nor could Jim even remember when he last made love to his wife. He believed his back trouble ended sex. And it seemed like years since he had played Nintendo with his children. His evenings and weekends were spent marooned in front of TV sportscasts, whiskey glass in hand.

Overweight from lack of exercise, Jim drank "to feel no pain." His cocktail hour started progressively earlier and he also grew increasingly dependent on painkillers. Too depressed to sleep, Jim turned to sleeping pills that left him groggy the next morning. Once, Jim spent two full weeks in bed, trying to "beat this thing." He felt so drugged he couldn't even concentrate on television. Not surprisingly, Jim grew antisocial and irrational.

Lonely and desperate

After years of solicitude, Jim's family and friends shunned his irritable and unpredictable manner. His children grew older and advanced in school and in their social lives without his involvement. His wife traded a part-time job for full-time employment, in part to escape from Jim and in part as a hedge against his possible unemployment. Lonely and increasingly desperate, Jim noticed that after continuous bed rest, his back hurt even more. Jim's worst nightmare, complete disability, was coming true.

Alarmed, Jim charged into battle against his pain, ever more determined to avoid defeat. He told himself he would never accept what was happening to him. Jim was at war with his doctors, his loved ones and, most importantly, himself. Jim became a splintered individual, with his once-coordinated mind and body now unglued.

An individual in as much pain as Jim finds mind and body do become disassociated, or split, by stress. Jim confronted his pain by trying to solve it, pushing futilely against the pain. Jim had reached an alarming stage of psychological confusion and spiritual emptiness. In all the advice he had garnered over the years, he had never learned about detachment, acceptance and transcendence.

Jim was certainly aware that he might lose his job, but he ignored the fact that he was perilously close to letting his family slip away as well. Overwhelmed by powerlessness and helplessness, he was both frightened and angered. Jim raged about the doctors' poor treatment. "They failed in their duty to take care of me," he argued. The tragedy was that Jim never mentioned his own duty to take care of himself.

After Jim's first visit to my chronic pain multi-disciplinary center, I knew that as long as he was unable to control his moods and emotions, or accept responsibility for his actions and decisions, he would remain in his present rut.

I immediately ordered a complete battery of physical work-ups and psychological assessments for an overview of his condition. I needed to determine how much of his pain was the legacy of his previous treatments. But I knew the most important factor in Jim's treatment would be his own attitude. Jim had the utmost confidence in doctors—who had given him more attention lately than did his family and friends. Still, after years of consultations, he was so confused by the contradictory medical advice that he could not make a decision, much less determine how to help himself.

I needed Jim's commitment

So many acute, pressing problems demand the attention of the healing professions. Historically, chronic pain has not been among them. Still, a doctor's deepest instinct is to provide comfort. The more I talked to Jim—and to hundreds of comparable patients—the more I understood that body affects mind and spirit, and vice versa.

Pain reverberated throughout Jim's life from office to bedroom. If I could find a way to lessen the pain in Jim's body or mind or spirit, I knew his distress would diminish in all three areas. Jim needed treatment with as many dimensions as his problems.

To formulate that treatment, I needed more than my medical books; I needed Jim's commitment. Jim unconsciously used his chronic pain to solve his myriad personal problems, unaware that his troubled mind and spirit set up conditions that kept him in pain. Changing Jim's attitudes and how he lived meant putting him back in charge of his body and behavior.

Patients like Jim, afflicted with chronic pain, need to hear, "There is no reason why you must suffer as you do." In the end, Jim's solution was within himself. But at first, Jim found this idea ludicrous.

Exercise: Identify the role pain plays in your life by answering these three questions, which I pose to all my patients at our first conference:

1. How would you describe yourself and your present situation?

2. What will you lose if you give up feeling and acting like someone in pain?

3. Aside from seeking pain treatments, have you tried to improve your life otherwise?

The day Jim described himself as, "Pretty much a failure, thanks to this back thing," he added, "What can I say? It's really taken over my life." Jim was surprised when I suggested that pain also provided benefits. Yes, good things came his way and Jim could avoid unpleasant tasks when he was an invalid. Jim had internalized the concept of secondary gains and learned helplessness.

Jim, for example, felt that his marriage had been suffering for some time, but couldn't say whether his back prompted his marital problems, or was a response to his marital problems. "It's a chicken-and-egg situation, Doctor," he confided.

Jim agreed he would be far happier if he could escape his pain and was eager to learn how. He knew that remaining an invalid destroyed his friendships and family life. "I'm certainly not very interesting any more," he admitted. "And I can't say I look great, either." These concessions were a step in the right direction, an important new approach to his own well-being.

Once Jim's clinical tests were available I persuaded him to enroll in a weight-loss program. Jim wanted to feel more attractive and admitted that "my big gut is straining my back."

However, he argued about my even more important recommendation—back school!

Back school

Back school is an intensive 5-hour course. It deals with mechanical stresses that can increase and exaggerate back pain and with exercises that decrease back pain. The course takes the responsibility for proper back care out of the doctor's hands and gives it to the patient, where it belongs. Back school is an educational process that gives a clear message: We have taught you all we know; now it's your responsibility to deal with it and get back to life again.

Yet this is easier said than done. For example, learning to stand and sit correctly is a sensible step, but Jim resisted meeting his quota of daily exercises.

Eventually Jim became enthusiastic about back school and the exercise program. Not only did he want to lose weight, but he wanted to lessen his need for painkillers. He didn't want to preach to his teenage children about the evils of drugs while he popped pills.

Like others with chronic pain, Jim had psychologically adapted to his suffering. I emphasized the importance of individual and family counseling along with good stress management techniques. Leery, Jim discussed my suggestions with his sister, a social worker, who agreed that counseling couldn't hurt. He admitted, "I don't know, Doctor. I'm not like my sister; I spend my life looking at columns of figures. I can't help thinking going to a shrink is probably voo-doo. But I'll give it a shot."

Giving up the gains

Although Jim had been hiding from his troubled marriage behind his pills and doctors' appointments, he realized that he loved his wife, and that unless they both overcame their difficulties, he would lose his marriage. Counseling sessions were one indication that Jim was now willing to sacrifice a secondary gain—hiding from a bad relationship—that pain offered.

Jim mentioned that when he encountered pain at work, he "tried to be Lou Gehrig—you know, grace under pressure." I explained that the worst thing he could do was to try to push away his pain. Since he was impatient and worried that the pain wouldn't pass, his muscles tensed and Jim felt even more pain. His helpless feeling grew, which in turn fed his already overwhelming image of himself as a failure.

> Jim's signs of spiritual blockage included tension, fatigue (no matter how much he rested), confusion and an inability to concentrate, whether on work or solutions to his situation. Jim avoided conflicts by staying in pain, feeling sorry for himself, and becoming totally reactive. Pain dictated his actions, thoughts and feelings. Just as his chronic pain changed his personality, it also radically altered his spiritual state and sense of self. I tentatively broached the idea that Jim needed to search his inner depths, detaching himself from the perception of pain.

> But the best way of coping, of detaching himself from his pain, was beyond Jim. Nothing in his upbringing or schooling had taught him that contemplation, self-focus and meditation could free him from his stress and chronic pain.

> I explained to Jim that some Eastern traditions emphasize the spiritual life, and suggested that he learn more about Eastern medicine and how it views illness as a process rather than a problem. I also urged Jim to investigate ancient Indian philosophers' notions of the spiritual journey one must undertake to recognize one's inner self. Jim could only argue that he was "no hippie" and wasn't going to "start following the Maharishi."

> Since Jim was an avid sports fan, I changed tactics and explained how athletes use imaging to improve their concen-

tration, motivation and self-esteem. Mental preparation can help an Olympic-class competitor see pressure as a challenge, rather than as a burden. Jim had to see his back pain exactly that way.

Jim slowly became intrigued with using his mind to transcend, if not cure, his pain. He also became more receptive to spiritual and other alternative methods and exercises, even experimenting with biofeedback and yoga for stress management. When he realized that he could change invisible autonomic bodily processes like tensing muscles and pulsing blood, he more willingly accepted that he indeed had an inner self, possibly affected by his pain. Jim was prepared to discover his true self.

Jim took the important step of meditating for introspection, then overcame his helplessness to the point where he could further expand his consciousness. To the deep relaxation he was learning through meditation he added self-imaging. Sketching the images from his dreams in a journal and using the techniques of Swiss psychologist Carl Jung, Jim began to understand the meaning of dreams and perceptions from his subconscious and unconscious. By understanding his spiritual self, Jim could repair his battered image. Jim's writing became a tool to record subconscious feelings and to find new meaning and direction for his life.

Dealing with chronic pain spiritually as well as physically and psychologically, Jim absorbed Jung's fundamental tenet: by experiencing life's conflicts directly and honestly, without avoiding or struggling against them, you will find that conflict holds the seeds of regeneration.

Jim was succeeding. His troubled, splintered self was coming back together. Allowing himself time to breathe deeply, meditate and self-visualize, he could reclaim his inner self. First, he abstractly understood his inner self; then, through his writing, he placed those feelings on paper, giving them tangibility and substance.

Such unified treatment can also enable you to take charge. You and your family will learn to face negative attitudes and secondary gains that perpetuate your pain. Of course there is no absolute cure for chronic pain, but you will reduce pain when you transform passive reliance on outside sources to active reliance on your own resources. And you will be able to recapture that sense of wholeness, the essence of life. You can feel healthy—even if your pain persists!

Pain is as personal as a thumb print,
a subjective experience we cannot measure objectively.

What is Pain?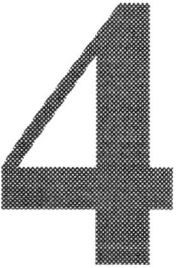

Pain is as personal as a thumb print. It is a subjective experience we cannot measure objectively. All of us think we know how much a backache or chest pain should hurt, but no medical test can yet detect pain or determine its severity. Chronic pain can indicate disease, signal an underlying condition, or both. Pain reflexes trigger far-reaching responses, with complex effects on your life and control over your behavior.

Pain is very real, whether or not its causes and effects are proven. Chronic pain is fed by physical (injury to back muscles), emotional (depression magnifies the effect of pain), and behavioral components. These three components affect our pain awareness. An overload in any one area will worsen chronic pain.

Pain is not static. It vacillates, improving and worsening over time in response to a multitude of internal and external stimuli. When you can identify and control these stimuli, you begin to recover. But you need essential information about chronic pain to gain control over your perceptions and sensations. Unfortunately, few physicians adequately explain pain to their patients.

Fear and anxiety, which inevitably accompany persistent, unexplained pain, produce tension and muscle spasm. When you become tense and anxious, your breathing and mobility are affected, which interferes with normal circulation. Poor circulation causes tissue swelling and nerve pressure, leading to more pain and heightened anxiety. This pain cycle gathers momentum as successive reactions gain in depth and intensity.

This chapter describes general neurological and physiological causes of pain. I discuss how your particular psychological, sexual and emotional makeup, as well as your social, ethnic and cultural background, contribute to pain perception: the sensory experience you interpret as pain. You will learn the specific exercises that change that perception.

Pain levels fluctuate with your internal and external relationships and environment. Change any one factor contributing to pain and you change the others. This alters the equation that measures your pain intensity.

Pain is not felt as pain until it passes from the point of injury, across your nerves, through the spinal cord and into your brain. Your pain circuits intersect with other circuits in the brain—emotional, sensory and awareness circuits. Thus, pain signals are interposed along other pathways, making all these pathways part of the pain circuit. You can see why pain must be fought in various ways.

Mind, body and chronic pain's vicious cycle

Unlike acute pain, chronic pain is not usually the symptom of something else. It is the problem, taking on its own identity, defying all cures and causing extensive changes in the sufferer's behavior and lifestyle. The individual's body, mind and spirit, all affected by intersecting pain circuits, are swept up in an escalating pain cycle that, like a weed, needs little nourishment to grow.

Debra

Debra, with severe jaw and neck pain, was victimized by just such a reverberating circuit. As Debra pursued our multi-disciplinary treatment program, her condition gradually reversed.

Debra tried pain control visualizations and felt less pain. Her visual images included green pastures and horses, because she had grown up in horse canyon country around Los Angeles, and recalled those times as pleasurable and relaxing. Debra's youth was filled with ponds, pastures and running brooks where she would spend endless hours. Now, in chronic pain, she drew upon those memories and images to help her escape her perception of pain. Eventually Debra became so adept at pain control visualization that her pain often subsided as soon as she lay down and closed her eyes. She would finish these exercises by projecting a future vision of herself in control of her pain and no longer its victim.

Understand the reverberating circuit and you too can trigger your body's self-healing abilities. You gain control of your thoughts and transcend the pain perception. Your intentions, desires and belief in recovery translate into physical healing.

These cycles are key to understanding your condition. The longer you've been in pain, the sharper your psychic anguish is likely to be. Sometimes you feel guilty: you believe your pain is the penance you deserve. Or you feel angry: your pain is the penance you **don't** deserve. Again, your emotional and physical states feed on each other. Uncertainty, impatience, anger, self-blame, helplessness and panic contribute to muscle tension, and spasticity, and more pain.

The medical literature has chronicled the link between mind and body. Research by Dr. George Engel, head of psychiatry at the University of Rochester, found four out of ten patients ascribed their chronic pain to emotional stress or depression. Most of the remaining patients who mentioned a physical event as the cause of their pain acknowledged some depression before the physical event occurred.

Much pain perception and response is learned. When we examine the development of pain engrams (specific response programs imprinted in the brain) we see that pain may be lessened by a systematic reprogramming of your pain response behavior. Dr. Ronald Melzack of McGill University Pain Center in Toronto helped establish the well-known and highly respected Gate Control Theory. It maintains that expectations of pain affect the pain experience by opening or closing the "spinal gate" mechanism. Opening the gate amplifies pain; closing the gate reduces it.

What happens to you physiologically when you feel pain? If you fall on a hard surface, the nerves located on the surface of your body become vigorously stimulated and send high-magnitude impulses along the nerve fibers into your spinal cord. They course through the spinal cord and ascend into the center of your brain. Here, in the portion of your brain called the thalamus, the pain transmission stops and is translated to a perception. What you perceive, according to the study, depends on what you have learned to expect. And those expectations can be altered with new learning. Further, your spinal cord and your midbrain can produce endorphins, the "wizard" chemicals that reduce pain by acting on the gate or on the brain, or on both.

Dr. Melzack demonstrated the learned pain response in an experiment with dogs in a restricted environment. Isolated as puppies, they did not learn the rules of social interplay among dogs or humans. As Melzack discovered, these dogs did not develop normal pain perception and sensitivity. He then duplicated these experiments with chimpanzees raised in a similar restricted environment. Both original groups returned to a painful stimulus over and over again, as if they had never been previously harmed. That is, they seemed to have no real perception of pain. We can conclude that development of pain engrams, or one's reaction to pain, is a learned behavior.

We program our brain responses by repetition and habit. Thus, when a similar subsequent event occurs, the program is activated and we react as we have in the past. Your pain experiences are similarly programmed into your brain's response system. When you experience pain, the perception and engram are reinforced in the nervous system and brain. Continue to think about pain and you allow that reverberating circuit to occur, reinforcing the pain perception.

If pain benefits you, perhaps enabling you to deny core feelings, preserve existing relationships or avoid a relationship you fear—you will have far more trouble succeeding in controlling your pain. The more you cling to pain as a coping mechanism, the more you will need psychological and spiritual support.

Exercise: Are there underlying reasons for you to hurt? Examine how your attitude toward pain may aggravate your pain.

1. Does chronic suffering hold real emotional advantages for you?

2. If you hurt less, will you lose something important to you? (For example, money in a legal case?)

3. Is your pain a way of mourning the loss of a cherished loved one?

Your family could be encouraging pain dependency. Family members too often "help" the chronic pain patient, doing for you what you must do for yourself.

Exercise: Write in your notebook the following statements. Then read them aloud four or five times a day, including each time you feel pain.

1. I will not talk about my pain with others—except within specific pain support groups or in family counseling sessions.

2. I will not use pain as an excuse not to perform important duties and responsibilities.

3. I will not let anyone aid me or do things for me I can do for myself.

4. I will not use pain to manipulate others.

5. I will not act helpless and hopeless. I will look positively upon life—after all, medical science has proven that it takes less energy to smile than to frown.

Physiological proof of how attitude and emotions affect pain comes from the body's own pain killers, endorphins and enkephalins. Research shows that laughter, exercise and other exhilarating activities help release these neurotransmitters into the body, unleashing their cargoes of morphine and opiate-like molecules. Conversely, negative emotions inhibit their release. There are at least three distinct endorphin-containing cells. All release peptides with opioid activity at their terminals, but they differ in distribution within the brain. The release of endorphins is the critical step in ending pain. However, researchers do not know when these specific pain-relieving systems activate nor to what extent they can alter pain behavior.

The brain is the source of all painkilling mechanisms, that is certain. While studying drug addiction, doctors Candace Pert and Solomon Snyder of John Hopkins University School of Medicine found that certain opium derivatives, such as morphine and heroin, would attach themselves to specific brain cells, much as a key fits into the right lock. Dr. John Hughs of the University of Aberdeen in Scotland isolated a chemical he name "enkephalin," which is similar to morphine and unlocks the brain's opiate receptors. When injected into the brains of rats, this chemical had a painkilling effect much like that of morphine or heroin. Endorphin, a variation of enkephalin, also is released by the pituitary gland. They are 200 times more powerful than morphine!

Speculation about endorphins continues. But you can learn to release endorphins yourself. You can regulate your autonomic body systems and thus control your own well-being. Your expectations of relief from chronic pain can stimulate your body to wellness by producing its own natural opiates. This regulates moods and reactions and makes the difference between peace of mind and anxiety; between hope and despair.

You see how the existence of neural networks that perceive pain have been established by anatomical, physiological and pharmacological mechanisms. The "wizard," the endorphin-mediated pain-modulating network, extends from the cortex of the spinal cord with major links throughout the inner workings of the brain. You can control pain-modulating systems in your brain by triggering your creative, spiritual and inner resources.

The notion that there are two kinds of pain—organic (real or physical) and non-organic (imaginary/psychogenic)—is nonsense. If something hurts, it's real. Our case histories underscore how the real/unreal dichotomy reinforces the tendency to isolate the patient's symptoms, thus foolishly focusing treatment on target organs rather than on the whole person. Instead of asking whether chronic pain is real, we should ask, "What factors influence it?"

Before the onset of chronic pain

Many of my patients are in good psychological health. Others have emotional difficulties. But generally, chronic pain does not simply happen. It expresses a mental, emotional or spiritual difficulty you are either ignoring or denying. If, like many pain patients, you have difficulty dealing with deepseated fear, anger or hostility, pain may have become your crutch for communication.

Whether or not you are in physical pain for psychological reasons, chronic pain always causes mental distress. Patients usually enter the pain cycle when they fear and resist pain. Chronic pain creates strong emotions. The entire cycle must be recognized and confronted if you are to acquire a positive attitude. Fearing pain only aggravates pain, and makes it a self-fulfilling prophecy.

The longer you have been in pain, the sharper your psychic anguish, especially if you are so disabled that you are now unemployed or, as happens too frequently, you are on your own or alienated from family members.

Exercise: If you believe you may be clinging to your pain, this exercise will be revealing: Talk to your pain. Sit quietly by yourself where you can feel comfortable and free from distractions. Close your eyes. Ask your pain whatever questions come to you. Some examples:

1. What payoff am I getting from you?

2. How am I using you?

3. Is there anything I avoid by having you around?

Answers to questions such as these will reveal thoughts and behaviors that underlie your pain. These habits cause you to suffer more than necessary. The chapters to come will show you how to replace old, harmful habits with new, beneficial ones.

A wonderful way to decrease fear is to write it away

Steps You Must Take Right Now   5

Remember the fable of the tortoise and the hare? The fable holds true in pain management: patients with the least promise often make the most progress.

Margot

An example is Margot, who approached her treatments with unbounded negativity. Margot was skeptical of the spiritual components of the program. She thought health care meant following her doctor's instructions. To my surprise, once she understood how the pain cycle works, she began to see how meditation and guided imagery might break up pain's reverberating circuit. Margot began to take control of her pain, tapped into her inner resources and was finally at peace with herself.

Margot's initial resistance to the spiritual path was rooted in her deep religious convictions: She believed that these two spiritual paths contradicted each other. Actually, the reverse is true. Margot's search for life's meaning occurred every time she looked beyond the superficialities of her life through her religion. Once Margot attempted relaxation, meditation and imagery, her resistance to the spiritual path vanished. Margot imagined the crippling joint pain in her hands melting away like ice on a hot summer's day. I was surprised at how easily Margot took to these techniques.

Studies by University of Pennsylvania psychology professor Dr. Martin Seligman and psychiatrist Dr. H.R. Hill prove that the more control people have, the less pain they suffer. Assuming responsibility for your own pain is a powerful, healthy response.

Unfortunately, chronic pain sufferers frequently feel trapped in a helpless abyss, ashamed and guilty about their condition and its repercussions. Chronic pain becomes the most important issue in their lives. They reorganize their schedules and regulate their behaviors to compensate for the extra pressures created by their pain. Their physical pain becomes their number-one concern. Because things don't get better quickly and their recovery is plagued with setbacks, they tend to exaggerate the possibility of lasting or permanent damage. The result? They fall into the helpless abyss.

Environment can dramatically affect your expression of pain and level of disability. Stress from chronic pain affects two environments: the external (the social, professional and family environment a person lives in) and the internal (the mental, emotional and physical condition of the sufferer). If the sufferer's pain is all-consuming, he has less energy to handle his environments. This lowered capacity to cope not only with the pain but with everyday responsibilities produces constant pressure, which is counterproductive to pain management

Behavior studies demonstrate that people can handle increasingly high levels of stress to an optimum point, after which coping mechanisms break down. Chronic pain significantly lowers your optimum point.

Exercise: Is your life permeated by fear? Most chronic pain sufferers would answer yes. Fear of the unknown makes you less productive and creative. A wonderful way to decrease that fear is to "write it away," listing in your notebook everything you fear due to chronic pain.

1. Explain the ways your chronic pain steals time from other activities.

2. List the ways pain perpetuates your procrastination.

3. Write the following phrase: "Time spent in pain, worried about how to handle it, is lost time."

4. Note some ways you can surmount your fears.

Remember that failure to manage your chronic pain with these exercises is not failure as a person. Undertaking the exercises in this book will bring you both success and failure. You cannot succeed at something unless you attempt it. Push through the fear and try something. Fear of failure only wastes energy.

Chronic pain compromises your ability to live effectively. What was once pleasurable becomes burdensome. You lose both physical and mental effectiveness. Chronic pain is indeed the great "un-coper." By reducing your problem-solving ability, it makes life difficult—sometimes seemingly impossible. Being able to write away your fears and come up with ways you can cope helps to clear away your sense of helplessness.

Exercise: By answering these questions you can determine how stressful your chronic pain is. Afterward, you will do a series of exercises to reduce your stress level.

1. Does your chronic pain make you feel irritable?

2. Do you lose patience with situations and problems that can't be readily solved?

3. Are you too impractical?

4. Do you drink more alcohol due to your chronic pain, or think alcohol will decrease the pain?

5. Do you take more drugs (prescribed and over-the-counter) due to increased pain?

6. Have you decreased your exercise and physical activities?

7. Have you decreased your sexual activity?

8. Do you isolate yourself from others because of your chronic pain?

9. Do you miss work more frequently?

10. Are life's problems piling up on you?

If you answered yes to five or more questions, you have a moderate to severe stress reaction caused by chronic pain. You must immediately reduce your stress and anxiety levels.

Irritability and impatience arising from your stress can be greatly reduced. Stop—whenever you find yourself losing patience or becoming irritable, stop. A pause breaks the stress-irritability cycle. Next, identify why you are irritable. Be specific. Write the reason in your notebook. Add some ways you might change the situation. To confront your irritability is effectively to grasp the situation. Immediate action gives you a sense of control over your chronic pain, which automatically reduces stress and anxiety.

Exercise: If you answered yes to questions 4, 5, 6, 7, 8 or 10, try this exercise: Plan one enjoyable activity for tomorrow. Write your idea in your notebook, along with the details for carrying it out. You now have something to look forward to. Next, list the activities and exercises you have enjoyed in the past. This is your reservoir of things to do when you feel down and out.

Exercise: If you answered yes to questions 2, 3, 9 or 10, you'll find this exercise helpful: When tasks seem overwhelming, simply break the great mass into small parts. Methodically attack each, proceeding to the next as soon as you complete the one before. This lessens your sense of being overwhelmed.

Never take life too seriously. Meeting every adversity and setback with grim determination can be grueling. Depression may be only a state of mind, but it affects the body. Laughter is one of the best remedies for depression. If you can laugh, you have one of the most powerful psychological antidotes for a slump. It's yours, free of cost, without a prescription and without danger of overdosing.

Accept some uncertainty. Tolerate some ambiguity. Meditation, relaxation, imagery and visualization exercises help you do this.

You can find lifelong peace, contentment and healing if you look for them. They are there for you if you decide you want them. On the other hand, if you look for negativity, you will find it in ample portions too. Which world you experience depends on what you look for. There is a direct relationship between what you get and what you think you deserve.

Exercise: Ask yourself two questions. Ponder the answers, and write specific responses in your notebook. Add all the details your imagination can muster.

1. If you could live your life over, what would you ask for that you didn't get in this lifetime?

2. What do you want now that you are not asking for?

Too much indulgence of self

Avoid isolation. Isolation is dangerous to your recovery. At first, being and feeling totally alone is a physical state, but it rapidly becomes a mental state. Soon you lose objectivity about your environment. You fear uttering words of despair, and it becomes more and more difficult to break the silence and communicate. This all leads to an "indulgence of self," which distorts your perspective and focuses awareness on your chronic pain.

Chronic pain causes constriction and rigidity of personality. It makes you one-dimensional. You become inflexible. You lack the resources to handle the full range of human stresses encountered in everyday life.

Add structure to your life. Design a routine of scheduled activities. Plan to be in certain places throughout your day. Do what you can to get something done.

Even if you answered yes to just one or two of the 10 questions above, practice the relaxation, meditation, creative visualization and imagery exercises in this book.

After diligently performing these exercises, you will gain a confidence that adds to your personality. Confidence means possessing sufficient internal resources to overcome adversity and prove equal to the task at hand. Confidence is linked to selfesteem; it is the belief that you can succeed and be proud of your accomplishments and yourself. Confidence and concern about the direction your life is taking indicate that you value the ups and downs of your life.

Good mental health integrates intense, and often conflicting pieces of your life and your personality into a comprehensive whole. It welds together these diverse elements into a complete self.

Goals

Few people plan their lives. Yet without an action plan you lack purpose in life. When you set a goal and approach it, you gain greater motivation and more self-esteem. Achievement of one goal strengthens your desire to achieve others. You attain a feeling of moving forward through life, and your sense of self-worth skyrockets.

Writing down your goals—where you want to go and what you want from life—makes them concrete and clear. You set the direction and path you choose to take. There is no magic in the real world! Life is choices. You must choose to make important changes in your life if you wish to heal your pain.

Exercise: This exercise sets goals. Answer these questions:

1. What activities do I want to do?

2. What activities would I like to do that I have stopped doing because of my chronic pain?

3. Where do I want to go with my life? Note: As you set long-term goals, also set sub-goals. If you select distant goals without short-term goals, your failure to see immediate progress will quickly discourage you. Achieving each sub-goal provides a sense of accomplishment.

4. What kind of life do I want after I recover?

5. What kind of individual would I like to be once my pain is gone?

Imagine that every thought you think, every word you utter, every feeling you experience will attract more of the same. Imagine that you can create the life you want to live by believing you already live it. The power to be an alive and multi-dimensional person comes from within!

As you tackle your goals, remember that less is more. That means don't overdo. Set daily goals just short of what you think you can achieve. If you exceed them you'll be quite pleased with yourself.

Warning: The moment you start feeling better, you may overreact because the contrast is so dramatic. You will want to be completely cured at once. But you're not completely cured. This is the time to pace yourself by performing precisely those goals you set for yourself. As we learned from the fabled tortoise, slower is faster! Hang in. Stick with your treatment. Get into the habit of taking things easy. Get out of the habit of pushing and straining.

Jim

Jim accomplished this. He put his troubled, splintered self back together by combining these components to whip the dreaded reverberating circuit. He re-acquainted himself with himself by spending less time drinking beer, watching television and burying his feelings. He replaced this destructive activity with time spent meditating. In the truest sense, this was Jim's first step toward recovery.

I instructed Jim to work on his feelings of powerlessness and helplessness by focusing on his past accomplishments and his future aspirations. He did just that, and slowly his sense of powerlessness diminished. He felt less like a victim of circumstance and more like a man running his own life. Jim began to view his pain as a challenge, not a burden.

Restore bodily functions

The joy of writing this book is in enabling you to tailor your own success program. You can adapt this program by learning how to reach within, carefully evaluating yourself, and structuring a program to emphasize your strengths. Powerlessness and helplessness can be overcome if you adapt my pain management program to your needs, using resources available right in your community.

There are many ways to restore bodily functions. They range from the passive modalities of heat, cold and electrical stimulation to active exercises for strength, increased range of motion, flexibility and relaxation. These exercises can be done at home. They are designed to increase your tolerance to sitting, increase your flexibility and strength, prolong your pain tolerance and prepare you to achieve full vocational restoration. This is where you actively manage you own health care. Once you know how to do these exercises and what range of motion your body can undergo, you can perform these exercises several times a day.

Debra

Like others with chronic pain, Debra believed activity would only increase her neck and jaw pain. She wore a brace at work and at home, keeping her neck in a rigid position. Debra was skeptical when I explained that this contributed to her neck pain. What she needed, I explained, was to increase her range of motion and flexibility. My physical therapist showed Debra exercises that would increase the range of motion and strength in her neck, shoulders and upper arms.

Occupational therapy focuses on the movements necessary for daily living and working. Again, you can control your pain. Let an expert show you the right exercises and educate you in the dynamics and physical structure of your body. Then examine how to make your work and home environment more user friendly.

> Debra noticed several things about her work and home that could be changed. Many of her activities at work contributed to her pain. For example, her chair and the height of her desk needed adjustment because the distance between the two caused her a great deal of neck and shoulder strain.

Learn to be well

Behavior modification and cognitive therapy also help you cope with pain. Behavior modification reinforces well behaviors and discourages pain behaviors. Cognitive therapy promotes positive ways to think and interact with others. Using behavioral techniques, you can arrange the contingencies (chances of things happening), rewards and punishments of your life to help you behave as you want to behave. You can exchange undesired behaviors for desired behaviors.

Instead of feeling tugged in different directions, you can take a deep breath and set your desired direction. Then go for it!

Even after identifying specific habits you want to change, you cannot always change by auto-suggestion, or by simply telling yourself to change. Yes, altering bad habits will give you a good feeling, a sense of control and increased self-esteem. But you'll need specific guidelines to genuinely and permanently change your life.

Change requires risk, but it is the first step to healing. Change is simply a break in your routine behavior. To heal, you must extinguish every behavior that impedes your progress and reinforces your pain.

Regardless of how maladaptive a lifestyle of pain and disability may appear, you will not relinquish that lifestyle unless you believe you can achieve a more successful lifestyle. But pain behaviors are learned behaviors. If you can learn to be disabled, you can learn to be well.

Exercise: These exercises help you change your routine behavior.

1. Stop thinking about your chronic pain. Thinking about it gives it power and control. You are too preoccupied with pain when a never-ending parade of thoughts centers around your suffering.

2. Turn negative pain thoughts into positive thoughts:

I can control my pain.

I am becoming more active.

I am constantly moving forward.

I can use breathing, relaxation, imagery, meditation and visualization to combat my chronic pain.

Thought stoppage

You maintain a bad habit by reinforcing it. You empower it by allowing it to take hold of you. You probably are not aware of how you are reinforcing bad habits. "Thought stoppage" enables you to detect patterns and express how you would like to act.

Exercise: Here are five very basic steps to achieve thought stoppage.

1. Sit in a comfortable chair.

2. Bring to mind one thought you want to control—perhaps your anxiety over your chronic pain.

3. As soon as the thought forms in your mind, say loudly, "Stop."

4. Next, say to yourself, "Calm."

5. Then relax the muscles throughout your entire body for five to ten seconds, bringing to mind a soothing or comfortable visual image.

Your aim? To break the destructive thoughts that wreak havoc in you. If you don't achieve that break, repeat the exercise and say "stop" longer and louder. Use thought stoppage as soon as unpleasant thoughts enter your mind and every time unpleasant thoughts enter your mind.

It's amazing how quickly you become aware of these thoughts. As soon as they flit through your mind, go through the "stop" routine, say "calm" and relax the muscles all through your body. You want that break! Additionally, you want to establish a counter-habit of eliminating negative thoughts. You do this through relaxation, visualization, imagery and meditation.

As with any habit, you must practice it at every opportunity. Perform this thought-stoppage exercise until it becomes automatic. Replace destructive thoughts with calming and relaxing visualization.

Thought stoppage is a simple yet effective technique you can use to stop anticipating chronic pain. And this allows imagery and visualization to work more effectively. How? You cannot think about two opposites at once. Your body cannot be both tense and relaxed. You can short-circuit the anticipation and dread of the pain and activate your built-in painkillers, the endorphins, whenever you put your mind to it.

Stop talking about your chronic pain to friends, family or whoever listens. Limit such discussions to your physician, psychologist or social worker and your pain support group. Otherwise, you must not discuss your chronic pain. Talking about it only gives it unwarranted power.

Remember: Focus on pain and your pain will increase. Focus on pain control and your pain will decrease.

Records and rewards

Monitoring yourself requires keeping records as a reinforcement. Self-monitoring changes your behavior. When you reward yourself for a certain behavior, the behavior pattern is fortified.

Exercise: Jot in your notebook the times when you most often talk about your pain.

Are you with a particular friend?

Are you with your spouse?

Are you under stress?

What time of day is it most likely to occur?

To summarize:

1. Stop "pain talk" right now.

2. Reward yourself for not talking about your pain.

3. Don't get upset with yourself if you make a mistake. Instead, try to figure out what went wrong. After you realize

what happened, do what you can to prevent the mistake from occurring again.

Cognitive therapy

Negative attitudes and feelings of helplessness make you feel out of control. The principles of cognitive therapy let you become more confident in your ability to manage your pain. This in turn allows you to distance yourself from external pain-solvers like medications and surgery.

Richard

Several years ago, Richard was injured while working in the warehouse of a large pharmaceutical company. The rollers of a heavy steel gate caught Richard, causing him to twist and fall on a concrete surface. Richard hurt his entire right lower extremity, especially his lower back. The sharp, dramatic twist caused tremendous muscle spasticity in his back and a bulging of one of his intervertebral disks. Predictably, Richard developed chronic pain in his back. Within the first year of the accident, he felt so much stress and agitation that he saw a psychiatrist and was placed on major tranquilizers.

In the beginning, Richard's sense of helplessness and despair simply demoralized him. But after 20 years of agonizing pain, Richard was tortured by muscle spasms, twitches and, most importantly, bitterness. Richard was angry, becoming the kind of person people avoided. Here was a man of 52 who existed in a hostile world, unable to see an escape.

The synergy of strong muscle relaxants, codeine pain killers and major tranquilizers left Richard moribund. His depression escalated, confining him to bed 24 hours a day, although he seldom slept. The lack of exercise caused atrophy, more muscle spasticity and contractures. Paradoxically, it was almost with a sense of pride that Richard pointed to his physical maladies: his right lower back, right leg, right foot. And he was an emotional wreck. His hands shook. His eyes blinked and twitched. His mouth moved in spastic grimaces.

Richard needed something to break the pain's reverberating circuit of physiological and psychological distress—not from the orthopedic surgeon he saw every month, nor the psychiatrist who prescribed tranquilizers. Nor was it going to be the family practitioner, unaware of all the medication Richard was taking. Neither could Richard's pain be eased by the workman's compensation lawyer Richard hired to "solve all my financial troubles."

If Richard was going to heal his chronic pain, he would have to stop giving away his power to people and things outside of himself.

Several important psychological elements affected Richard's pain management. Richard lacked introspection. Before entering the chronic pain multi-disciplinary program, he was unaware of how his demoralized attitude affected his life. He didn't bother to examine and search, and thus failed to reach out to some wonderful inner resources that were his to tap.

What was so fascinating was Richard's potential. He had all the secrets within him; he just didn't know how to put them to use. Although he was sensitive, his outward anxiety and hostility masked his caring and loving. Accepting his spiritual dimension became his focus, transforming his anger into acceptance and serenity.

But until Richard made that inner journey, only despair and hopelessness surfaced, and that became his world. Richard was not to blame; he was not a "bad" person. Working with Richard was simultaneously difficult and rewarding: Difficult because the way he handled and coped with pain was destructive. Rewarding because every session with Richard was an adventure, a fresh look at the marvels of life, specifically at an individual who withholds from himself all his wonderful resources.

I knew that Richard's attitude was crucial. As he became a full participant in his multi-disciplinary program, he learned to replace medication with psychological exercises. This made him the pain manager and placed him on the road to healing. He learned the value of "self-talk," and taught himself to relax. He learned to view situations more positively and constructively by thinking things through before feeling the pain. He learned to convert negatives into positives. Thinking things through and talking to himself allowed him to create the emotions he wanted to feel. Through self-talk, Richard found he was capable of ordering himself to act in a rational, non-demanding way.

Richard is a fine example of how cognitive therapy with assertion training can handle chronic pain.Once he understood the role psychology plays in life, Richard began to take an active role in his pain control.

As you continue reading, you are going to be excited by the possibilities of self-recovery. Not only does my program challenge you mentally and physically, but it stimulates you to change your philosophy toward life! You are recovering your body and soul. What a marvelous sensation!

These experiences teach you to accept your feelings: To look at them and deal with them, rather than punishing your body by holding feelings in. You already know how pent-up feelings hurt you physically. They are never laid to rest until you accept and deal with them.

Listen to yourself and how you feel about a particular situation. When you unleash those feelings you reduce the chance that distress and suffering will settle into your back or neck. When you think through a situation, know how you feel about it and then act in an assertive, productive way, you become successful at controlling the forces around you.

Work now to change your way of life. Besides practicing new ways of dealing with feelings you once suppressed, you can continue exercises that help produce physical relaxation—even when emotional stress cannot be avoided.

Detach from your body

Practicing creative visualization is one way to tap into your unconscious. Creative visualization fosters detachment from the body and frees you to go beyond your pain.

Exercise: Try a learning-through-doing exercise. Imagery activates endorphins, the body's built-in painkillers. Breathing is a crucial first step to imagery, creative visualization and relaxation. No longer will you take short, shallow breaths. You will breathe long and deep.

Take a deep breath.

Let it out slowly.

Close your eyes.

Your arms and legs are heavy and warm.

Your heartbeat is calm and regular.

Your breathing is deep and regular.

Focus your attention on your breathing. Sense the cool air coming into your lungs as you breathe in, the warmth as you exhale. As you experience the calm, deeply relaxed sensations of each inhalation, visualize oxygen traveling down into your body.

Your goal is to attain total body relaxation within 20 seconds, and to maintain that relaxation for two minutes. When relaxation is achieved this quickly, it can pre-empt pain responses before they get started.

Imagination is the key. It is your ability to create ideas or pictures in your mind. In creative visualization you use your imagination to create a clear image of something you want.

Richard wished to become a happy, open, productive and creative person. He had many inner resources, such as a sardonic wit and a dramatic flair, that could be put to new uses. He began to visualize himself as someone with a vibrantly healthy body, free from pain and able to run on the beach and dance. This visualization of himself as young, strong and healthy encouraged him to perform more activities. Better yet, he could no longer sustain his image as a man with a serious disability, unable to engage in physical and emotional activities. The two were incompatible.

Utilizing your imagination involves exploring, discovering and changing your deepest, most basic attitudes. Meditation can achieve this even more powerfully. It puts you in touch with your inner self—a wellspring of love, peace, strength and creativity. From that place, you can transcend your pain.

The ideas in this chapter will help you believe in yourself and your ideas. In later chapters you will learn other ideas, different exercises. Then you can decide which of these techniques best suits your pursuit of good health.

Unusual as it sounds to Americans,
opening to your pain is opening to life.

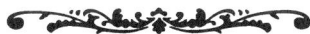

The Power of Acceptance 6

Chronic pain is often subconsciously used to protect against more difficult problems. This is a common but seldom recognized cause of chronic pain. But what we do subconsciously and unconsciously cannot be undone. This book teaches how to reach your subconscious and unconscious.

Unusual as it sounds to Americans, opening to your pain is opening to life. Eastern philosophy teaches that awareness of pain leads to natural transformation. The alternatives, which consistently fail, are forced change and active resistance.

Forced change and forced control simply do not work. The flexible tree that bends with the wind survives. The rigid tree does not. Using meditation, the relaxation response, creative visualization and imaging, you can become that flexible individual. You open yourself to new ways of thinking, feeling and being.

You realize that your pain does not define you. You are much more, much greater than your pain. Thinking and feeling positively by creating images and visualizations will be a new way for you to experience chronic pain.

Richard

After years of fighting lower back pain, Richard finally allowed himself to contemplate his pain through a deeply relaxing meditation technique that concentrates on breathing. He began daily meditation that emphasizes visualizing very pleasant sensations. Richard's mind placed him on a snow-capped mountain, or on the ocean's waves, or in the middle of a gurgling brook. Richard became calmer, more alert and less tense. "My back still hurts," he said, "but it bothers me less." Pain was no longer all consuming.

Relinquishing your resistance to pain does not mean giving up. It means experiencing pain without superimposing on it needless judgments, blame and self-hatred. Chronic pain unleashes a Pandora's box of guilt, anger and other negative emotions. Richard, for example, had an overwhelming sense of responsibility. When the relentless pain kept him from fulfilling all of his "I shoulds," he criticized himself mercilessly.

The paradox is that the more we try to control life, the less control we have. The serenity prayer from Alcoholics Anonymous is a good reminder of this:

> God, grant me the serenity to accept the things I cannot change,
> the courage to change the things I can,
> and the wisdom to know the difference.

Relief came only when Richard realized that his physical suffering was a messenger from his own consciousness. He was "resisting a rest." He needed to be quieter and more introspective. He needed to stop driving himself. The answer to pain and grief is to accept it and flow with life.

Life is as you see it

Throughout your life you have witnessed the interplay between inner and outer, between structure, form, function and content. Now you must go beyond, to learn that you can change a situation by changing how you look at it. An ancient yogi says, "Life is as you see it." The Yogasutras of Patanjali, an ancient guide to spiritual practice, states, "Yoga is the stilling of the modifications of the mind."

You can achieve awareness of the mind. What you think can be a choice rather than a habit. Your pain can be a vehicle for transforming how you view your life and the world.

Consider the amazing achievements of individuals with severe disabilities. Cambridge physicist Stephen Hawkings and Irish painter and writer Christy Brown are two examples. The one characteristic that is found in each's success? Passion. Each has an unrelenting persistence in achieving something they believe in. Make healing your pain your passion, and your conduit to a new perspective on life.

Your answers to this Attitude Questionnaire will help you clarify your current attitudes about pain and life. Answer these questions True or False.

1. My pain is excruciating.

2. I have learned to live with my pain.

3. I still have pain, but not as much.

4. I get more and more tense all the time.

5. I'm not letting little things upset me.

6. I'm discouraged, depressed and have nothing to look forward to.

7. There are few things in life that give me pleasure.

8. People no longer want to hear about my pain.

9. I've been feeling run down lately because I never get a chance to relax.

10. My life has become unmanageable.

11. I have a sense of connection with my inner self.

12. I have an idea of where I'm going.

13. My relationship with my family is a good one.

14. Sometimes I get angry at seemingly unimportant things.

15. I need something more to fulfill me.

16. I don't see any end to all this pain.

Date this questionnaire and answer these questions again in three months, after mastering breathing, creative visualization, imaging, relaxation and meditation. You will notice striking differences. Pain is the call of your soul for recognition. The exercises in this chapter are direct ways of responding to your unconscious and subconscious.

Don't just read the following exercises; do them. You may need to perform them several times a day. You'll find that your sense of accomplishment will increase and, with it, your self-esteem.

Exercise: One quick way to become receptive to denied feelings is to sit quietly, close your eyes and become aware of your breathing. Conscious breathing enhances your understanding of the interconnection between external and internal worlds. When you feel anxious, tense and fearful, you breathe shallowly. This is one way your body keeps feelings at a distance.

Begin this exercise by becoming aware of the shallowness of your breathing. Then concentrate on deeper and slower breaths. Sitting still, letting go of your anger and concentrating on the way you breathe will serve as your transformation. Immersing yourself in your deep breathing allows your feelings to surface and enables you to respond. Subconsciously, your breathing mirrors how you feel and what you are experiencing. Like the flexible tree in the wind, your mind can bend and challenge your denial.

Deep breathing initiates relaxation. Moreover, deep breathing helps you overcome fatigue by increasing your oxygen intake and expelling carbon monoxide along with other metabolic wastes. Breathe deeply and your mind will begin to wander, drifting toward more pleasant feelings and thoughts.

Laura

Laura found that, instead of resisting difficult and hurtful feelings stemming from childhood sexual and physical abuse, she could, with deep breathing, accept those feelings as part of herself. By accepting and forgiving, Laura reached a higher level of consciousness. Her concentration on breathing broke the reverberating circuit and replaced it with a cycle of deep breathing, relaxation, imaging and creative visualization. Gradually she freed herself of the anger and hostility from her past. Her new perceptions and sensations created new attitudes.

Laura learned that the more she pushed away her rage over the physical and sexual abuse, the more vigorously it would swing back and knock her flat on her back in pain. It was only when she breathed deeply, relaxed, meditated and moved through these feelings, however difficult, that she transformed her pain into a continuum of inner and outer growth. It became a constant expansion and contraction—just like the eternal breath.

Laura came to terms with her feelings, channeled them constructively and acknowledged the negatives as well as the positives. As she moved into, through and beyond her pain, Laura opened herself to new possibilities. From her new perspective, pain was no longer the all-consuming factor.

Clearly, a key to healing is unlocking paralyzing repressed feelings of grief and pain.

The direct route to meditation

Relaxation is the simplest, most direct route to meditation. The best beginning exercise I know comes from *The Relaxation Response* by Dr. Herbert Benson of Harvard Medical School. In it he writes of his success in the use of relaxation for the treatment of hypertension. He also explains the philosophy and scientific foundation for using relaxation exercises to relieve physical, mental and emotional tension.

Benson's relaxation technique is compatible with all spiritual and philosophical beliefs. I claim no innovation, but simply state that this tried and tested method works. Dr. Benson suggests this:

Find a place free from distractions, such as a quiet room. Make sure the area has only dim light. This fosters peace of mind. Sit in a comfortable position free of undue muscular tension. If you lie down, there is a tendency to fall asleep. Various postures of kneeling, swaying or sitting in a cross-legged position are advised.

Close your eyes. Concentrate on an imaginary spot and try to clear your mind of all outside thought. Focus your mind on an object, perhaps a silently repeated word like "one," "love" or "ohm." Repeat this word over and over again in the same way. Attention to the normal rhythm of breathing is useful and enhances the repetition of the sound or word. As you breathe out, say the word or sound. Breathe in. Breathe out and say the word. Remember to breathe deeply and slowly from the diaphragm, saying the word with each expiration. Continue in this fashion, dismissing intrusive thoughts as they come, for 20 or 30 minutes.

You will begin to feel free of tension and quite relaxed. Adopt a let-it-happen, passive attitude, witnessing whatever thoughts and imagery drift into your awareness. With your eyes closed, maintain deep relaxation of all of your muscles. Breathe through your nose. Permit relaxation to occur at its own pace; the breathing will foster this. Practice this relaxation exercise, with no thought to how well you're doing. As time goes on you will become more skillful with it. Allow yourself the time and the freedom to learn how to relax; learn to accept and welcome a fixed period of time without distractions or interferences.

You are learning to relieve anxiety, stress and tension by replacing those emotions with ones that help you achieve inner peace. You come away from this calm feeling renewed and refreshed, your body musculature limbered and relaxed. You have gained confidence that you can break up the strangulation on your musculature that tension and stress cause. As you learn the basic workings of your body and see how you have regained control over them, you no longer feel helpless and hopeless. Your approach to life is now based on "I can."

Deep muscle relaxation is not only a refreshing experience but the first step in production of the body's own painkiller. You will learn to control and relax even the smallest muscles in your body and, in this relaxed state, mental imagery can foster endorphin production. Without first practicing relaxation, imagery messages are blocked and never reach the brain's control mechanisms. Relaxation allows your body to be in harmony, which opens you to the body's interconnected channels.

Slowly, you are beginning to understand how the mind, body and spirit interplay with one another.

When you use relaxation techniques, certain physiological changes occur within your body:

1. Oxygen consumption is reduced; less energy is required to run your body.

2. The amount of carbon dioxide expelled decreases.

3. Respiration rate is reduced and your body conserves energy.

4. Blood flows more freely through expanded vessels.

5. Pulse rate drops 10 percent.

6. Blood pressure drops 10 percent.

7. An overall sense of well-being ensues.

8. Your ability to produce endorphins increases.

Now it's time for you to attempt a relaxation exercise. Begin by warming up. As discussed above, inhale deeply, close your eyes and hold your breath for three seconds. Then exhale slowly, silently repeating a simple, meaningless word. At the end of the exhalation, the abdomen should be moderately contracted. Repeat this procedure five times. Each time you breathe out, notice the slight sag in your body, as though it is sinking. Let this happen. Do not force anything. The first few times you attempt this exercise, you might feel you have made no progress. Do not give up. Soon you will accomplish your goal: relaxation.

Remember, you can never rid yourself of all of the tension in your body. Some tension is essential to maintain attention, body structure and daily performance. What you are getting rid of is the excess tension that cultivates chronic pain.

Examine your muscle tension, starting at your feet and working toward the top of your head. Be aware of any tight muscles. As you reach your shoulders, observe the muscles of the back and sides of your neck and your jaw. Again, take a deep breath and let your body sink as you exhale. Do not let your arms touch the sides of your body; keep your legs slightly apart. Let your jaw sag. Relax the muscles in your face.

When part of your body is injured or starts to hurt, it instinctively responds with muscle tension. The muscles around the injured part tense. The ability of your muscles to go from a tense to a relaxed state is important. Learn to "will" tension and relaxation, and you are in full control of the physical and mental components of your body. Start by tensing a particular muscle group so that you learn to recognize the symptoms of tension. Hold the tension for five seconds. Now relax the tightness in that particular muscle.

You may have a high degree of muscle tension without being aware of it. You have been so tense for so long that the tension is normal. You have forgotten what it feels like to be relaxed! This exercise produces relaxation in a group of muscles and teaches you what different levels of tension feel like.

Exercise: This exercise combines progressive muscle relaxation with the imagery processes.

1. Focus your thoughts on your right hand. Form a mental picture of your hand. Make a fist, squeezing tightly, and hold the pressure for ten seconds. Now let go. Let your fingers spread outward, releasing all the tension. As you unclench your fist, you will feel a tingling sensation in your hand. This is tension being released from the muscle.

2. Now tense the muscles in the back of your neck and your

shoulders. Hold the tension for ten seconds and let go. Notice that your neck and shoulders feel heavy—even warm—as you relax your body.

3. Now do the same with the your lower back and hips. Tense the muscles, hold it for ten seconds and let go. Can you feel the tension flowing from the very center of your lower back?

4. Now tense all of the muscles along your spinal muscula- ture, from your neck, through the middle portion of your back, to the lower back. Hold for ten seconds and let go. You will feel enormous relief as you release the tension you cre- ated along your spinal musculature.

Practice these exercises at least once a day. But also learn to check your muscle tension periodically to make sure it is not building up. At regular intervals throughout the day, take a minute or so to check for signs of tension. Consciously relax those muscles. Keep your body as relaxed as possible at all times. Eliminate all unnecessary muscle tension.

Exercise: This creative visualization exercise transcends the pain. Set aside some special time for this exercise. Go to your quiet place, where no one and nothing can interrupt you. Sit com- fortably on the edge of a bed or chair, spine straight and balanced. A straight spine helps the energy flow. Watch how your breath goes in and out, and breathe more and more slowly as you relax the muscles in your body. Each calm, slow breath breaks the ten- sion in your body. Count backwards from 20. As you breathe deeply and more slowly, you will relax more and more.

Imagine the tension being released with each exhalation, flowing down your body from your head to your feet. As you inhale, imagine gathering more tension from within your body and letting it flow out from top to bottom. Relax each muscle in your body, letting tension flow out with each exhalation. Now imagine the tension pooling at your feet in the form of energy, and let it bubble slowly up through the center of your body and out the top of your head like a fountain of light. Then it flows down the outside of your body to your feet.

Imagine that you are in some idyllic country setting, perhaps relaxing on soft green grass beside a cool river; or meandering through a beautiful, lush forest; or alighting on a snow-capped mountain. Choose a place where you have been, or where you would like to go. Visualize the details. Create it any way you like. You have total control over your imagination!

Now pinpoint the exact center of your pain and visualize a radiant, warm light within it. Feel it spread and grow, shining out from you until, like a golden sun, you radiate loving energy on everything and everyone around you.

Say to yourself, "Divine light and divine love flow through me and radiate from me to everything around me." Repeat this to yourself until you have a strong sense of your own spiritual energy.

End this visualization on a positive thought, known as an "affirmation." You are merging the conscious with the subconscious and unconscious. Each time you make an affirmation, you allow a positive vision of change to seep through to the deepest levels of your mind. It is crucial to make this visualization very enjoyable, and to conclude with a positive statement.

In the next chapter you will learn how to spiral through your own center, discovering your inner self and combining the inward and outward parts of your consciousness. Like Laura, you will learn how to reflect upon and move through your past experiences.

*Because you see no answer from
where you are does not mean there is no answer.*

Looking Within

7

Imagine that Humpty Dumpty is a deep and complicated person, more a three-dimensional puzzle than a hollow shell. What if some of his inner pieces were mislaid? Could Humpty be put back together again? I think not. This chapter is about restoring the inner pieces you have mislaid.

Like most sufferers, you probably find the sense of helplessness that accompanies chronic pain overwhelming and exhausting. You probably feel little or no inclination to improve your situation. The notion of drawing on your inner resources seems ludicrous when your overriding emotion is a sense of being drained. Yet experience has taught me that the only way to repair the damage chronic pain does to your self-image and create a mindset that allows you to live with—even conquer—pain is to draw on your inner resources. Cultivate your spirituality. To begin the journey out of meaninglessness, you must affirm life.

Your attitude toward life determines how meaningful your life will be. According to Eastern philosophy, "The dynamic process of growing is envisioning oneself as being more than the parts that make up the whole." All psycho-physical realities, including one's body, feelings, perceptions, consciousness and volition, are in a constant state of flux, according to Eastern philosophy:

In my journey/I suffer from sickness/
And yet my dreams/Are running in withered fields.

In addition to their physical pain, my patients are usually in spiritual pain, unaware of the intricate workings of their inner selves. Many refuse to accept the need to look within, but pain can turn on your inner light. An awareness of what is within can propel you upward emotionally and spiritually, irrespective of what is happening to your body. This is true transcendence.

You may be so immersed in chronic pain that you have no idea how to get out. But because you see no answer from where you are does not mean there is no answer. It means only that you do not see it. There is an answer—a way to heal your chronic pain, a way to control the suffering and discomfort it causes. And it will come. Relax. Meditate. Visualize yourself bathing in a lake's warm, calm waters. Do something you enjoy. The answer will appear in its own way and its own time. Be patient when you feel stuck. If you panic, you will fall into a sea of turbulent anxiety and lose all the peace you have worked so hard for.

Challenges that immobilize you can be opportunities to find the strength within you that is begging to come out. It takes time and patience. As you peel away your disillusions like an onion's skin, your sense of fulfillment will never seem greater. You will find that all the strength and all the answers you ever need come from within.

Beyond the conscious mind

Psychoanalyst Carl Jung pointed out that all ills stem from identifying only with our conscious knowledge, ignoring the deeper levels of our being. Cut off from our source of strength and yearning for wholeness, we suffer anxiety, fear, tension depression. Jung stressed that psychological wholeness blends psychology and spirituality, and creates no boundaries between mind and soul.

Jung bridged Eastern philosophy and Western psychology with his concept of the unconscious—a world he considered as vital and real a part of our lives as the conscious mind and ego, yet infinitely wider and richer. The unconscious is at once a cache of personal wisdom and creativity and a cauldron of personal fears and discontents. The language of the unconscious is symbols, and one of its methods of communicating with you is your dreams. Becoming aware of your unconscious symbols will help you achieve inner balance and provide powerful insight into the role of pain in your life. It is never a matter of chance when a person has chronic pain.

Jung found that the core of Eastern teachings consisted of looking inward to the mind. This, he believed, is the source of our self-liberating power. He became convinced that we must seek values within. But as Jung acknowledged, "People will do anything, no matter how absurd, to avoid facing their own souls."

Jung believed that images come to your awareness from all parts of your psyche (your center, self or soul). Jung felt that every human being has a craving for a rich inner life. He also believed that this drive for self-awareness was tied to an urge to connect with something larger, something more than your own physical being.

Now, working from Jung's concept, do this: Visualize a relaxing beach scene. As you do, your body relaxes exactly as it would on a real beach, because your unconscious and your autonomic systems do not distinguish between real and imagined. Simply by repeating an image like the relaxing beach scene, you can reach your higher self.

Next, relax and think about something totally removed from your present surroundings. Imagine yourself in a whirlwind of soft, warm, comfortable breezes. Or place your mind, body and spirit on a mountaintop where you are camping. You are lying in high grass under the big sky after a long hike. Lose yourself in this picture for several minutes.

By understanding your soul or center, the collective unconscious, you can achieve your inner transformation. Your unconscious is like a mixed terrain of mountains, lakes and forests. But the unconscious is night. While it is the source of all inspiration, creativity and wisdom, you cannot see it.

Suppose, though, you light a fire in a specific spot. Suddenly you can see the mountains, lakes, forests and so on. That fire is consciousness. Nevertheless, the unconscious, speaking in the language of symbols, is the guide that will point the way to your destination. You can transform what is within to the level of your consciousness through relaxation, meditation, imaging and creative visualization. Eastern philosophy clearly states that when the conscious mind is clear and unobscured, it is the root of happiness, liberation and bliss. This, the highest state of consciousness, is known as "clear light."

There is nothing esoteric, mystical or strange about experiencing other levels of consciousness. We meet our unconscious mind every night in our dreams. Jung found confirmation of his theories in his patients' dreams. You experience your unconscious every time you become immersed in the moment. For example, when a glorious sunset wipes your mind clear of other thoughts, or you awaken from a deep, dream-filled sleep, you feel cleansed, restored, blissful, transported by an array of exquisite feelings. You are aware of what was always there.

Both Jungian and Eastern meditation are concerned with the disoriented individual. The aim of meditation is to help the suffering man restore his balance, making the illness (in this case, chronic pain) an opportunity for growth by training the mind to remain calm. It does not matter how long you have had chronic pain; you can make a complete reversal in the process whenever you choose. Simply look deeper. Ask yourself these questions:

1. How can I be happier?

2. How can I get more out of my life?

3. What is it I want out of life but believe I cannot obtain?

4. Is there a difference between how I live with my chronic pain and how I wish to live once I start to heal?

5. What is my next step on the road to healing?

6. How can I arrive at that deeper level?

Jung envisioned that the self could control the body and the mind and, thus, control the outer world. That is a key concept: Your own self can be the mechanism that controls your body and mind, and thus transcends your perception of pain. Your outer world can be rearranged by the inner workings of your soul.

Tapping the unconscious

Focusing on your unconscious was part of Jung's groundbreaking work. Your personal unconscious comes into existence through your experiences. This is universal to us all. For Jung, this collective unconscious was seen as the depth of the self.

While Jung did not study chronic pain specifically, he was very interested in physical illness. He once made an accurate medical diagnosis after listening to a patient's dream. He stressed synchronicity, the link between physical and psychological states, observing that, "The physical disorder appears as a direct mimetic expression of the psychic situation." As he studied our relationship with our unconsciousness, he recognized that pain and illness could disassociate us from our spiritual life, and that physical healing had to be accompanied by a restoration of inner harmony.

Jung used the concept of "doing inner work" to describe looking inside oneself for insight and peace of mind through reflective skills such as dreamwork, meditation, imaging and visualization.

Jung's thought provides a particularly effective basis for dealing with the spiritual repercussions of chronic pain. If you have been in pain for a long time, you need inspiration to help you out of your suffering. Jung believed that your unconscious harbors not only your deepest desires and fears, but your strongest hopes for fulfillment. There is the opportunity for a sudden burst into consciousness of a process worked through in the subconscious. This sudden beam of light can electrify a turning point in your life.

Listed below are techniques based on Jung's work on summoning possibilities and hopes. Each technique places responsibility on you. Your responsibility motivates you to take physical and emotional well-being into your own hands. Thus, your control of your pain becomes closely related to your attitudes and actions. To be in control of this interaction requires a practiced sensitivity and response to the needs of body and mind. Jung stressed this psycho-physical oneness of all life.

Keeping a dream journal

Our dreams often pinpoint our problems and offer solutions. Before you go to sleep, tell yourself you will remember your dreams in the morning. Chances are that you can be successful in recalling parts of them. Keep a pad and pencil by your bedside and write down your dreams as soon as you awaken.

Even if you do not fully understand your dreams, you will learn something from reading your notes and will soon sense their importance. This in turn will lead to an attempt by your unconscious and subconscious to produce healing. You might even consult a therapist skilled in dream interpretation.

Exercise: When you awaken in the middle of a dream, write down what you remember. Then complete it as you desire, letting your imagination flow freely. You will be interspersing the unconscious with the conscious. Even though you might not consciously understand the dream, it will help you define a new level of awareness and uncover new meanings to life.

Writing to find yourself

Reminiscing serves a purpose. It lets you adapt and prepare psychologically for the next phase of your life. A daily journal enables you to make your reminiscence more conscious, deliberate and enjoyable. Keeping a daily journal reconnects you with all parts of your life and provides you with the inner thread of your life's movement. This unfolding process is an opportunity to discover life's inner meaning. When you discover the meanings and symbols from your life and put them into words, you transform self-destructive feelings into a creative act. You are at the helm and can direct these feelings and thoughts.

Writing is an active process, and whenever you act you regain control. Don't get bogged down and be concerned with your writing ability. Just be willing to write down your feelings as part of the process. When you write a daily journal, you begin to explain unexplained patterns.

The following exercise helps you mobilize your feelings and turn off your logical mind. Dump the thoughts. Fill the pages with your perceptions and sensations. This is a crucial exercise that combines deep breathing with writing.

Exercise: Take a long, deep breath. Imagine your stomach literally digesting your thoughts and the logic that interferes with your feelings. You want those interfering thoughts to be ripped to shreds by your digestive juices.

Focus on your breathing. Like a Buddha, inhale and let your stomach expand. With each long, deep breath, you allow your sensations and perceptions to permeate through your blood—to each artery and vein—and diffuse your whole system.

Now begin to write. Think of writing as breathing: the first step is to inhale deeply and let the flow of your body's inner workings guide your writing. Allow your subconscious and unconscious to control your writing. Do not stop that flow. Do not allow thoughts to interfere with the process. Rather, feel your way through this...and write!

Continue to do this for a specific time, your "designated time to write," which should last at least 30 minutes. Make allowances in your schedule to do this exercise at least twice a day. This way you are constantly in touch with your inner feelings.

This process allows you to write as a whole being. Your entire body is perfused with the nourishment of your deep breathing. Your body is full of your feelings, perceptions and sensations. This is the point where your subconscious, unconscious and conscious coalesce, making you whole. As the deep breathing exercise prepares you to write about your feelings and perceptions, also utilize the other exercises: meditation, relaxation and imaging. Your previous feelings of disconnection will be transformed to a mind of clear perceptions.

You cannot comprehend the rhythm of your life as you go through your everyday existence. Whereas before it was easier to see outside yourself, now, through these exercises, you can delve inside yourself. You chip away at the external to connect with your inner self. Eventually those actions, feelings and thoughts that you did not understand begin to make sense.

When you begin writing, focus on your immediate emotions—your environment in that moment. You'll discover that your writing gains tremendous energy, and you'll be able to write despite your pain. Writing allows you to release your pain the same way discussing your pain in chronic pain groups does. You'll soon discover that writing permeates your life in may ways. As you write you are providing detailed information about your feelings and thoughts. Thus, writing is a constant source of vitality and life.

Writing also allows you to feel out your situation and break through. When you write, you delve into the world of your feelings. You wander through this new world and discover various shapes and sides of yourself. At the end, when you come back to "reality," you realize that you are carrying a new message about your chronic pain. Writing allowed you to lose control, step out of your ordinary world, see new perspectives, and learn that things can change. Nothing is so solid or so structured that it cannot be changed and transformed.

Connect with your senses when your mind flashes on something. This first flash is the immediate world of your feelings, before your thoughts censor and criticize. Writing helps you blast through your internal censor to capture your basic perceptions. Use your writing to pull to the surface that which is submerged and repressed.

This is freedom. It permits you to know who you are. It means understanding what you want to do in the short span called life, and then doing it. All of life's experiences, memories and feelings are within you. Writing lets you reach deep, grab them and bring them to the surface.

Writing can be simple: Let go of everything and just write. Allow yourself to be awkward. You are stripping yourself. You are exposing your life and recording your thoughts and feelings as they roll through your mind and leap onto your journal pages.

This is how breathing and writing are linked. Boundaries disappear in these processes. The origin and creation of your writing is your unconscious and subconscious. The same is true with deep breathing. You give yourself free space to breathe, explore and express your feelings. You begin to believe in something below the mind's surface. It is the next layer, like those layers of the onion. You must believe there is something real below the surface of your life.

But it takes time. Don't become frustrated. You need perspective for your feelings to sift through your consciousness. Trust that you will gain this perspective. Through your writing you will embrace life and trust your own mind, body and spirit.

As you write in your journal, you will be amazed at how much resistance you face. This is because you are expressing feelings and ideas you have avoided for years. Now they are emerging through your writing. This is your chance to look at the inertia, insecurities, self-hate and fear that contribute to your chronic pain.

Anything we do fully is a journey alone. You can't expect others to match the intensity of your emotions or to completely understand what you are feeling. Still, it need not be a lonely process; you are communicating with your inner self.

Exercise: In addition to writing 30 minutes twice a day, do this next writing exercise. It takes 5-10 minutes three times a day. I suggest morning, mid-afternoon and evening. Express wishes that float around in your mind, thoughts you don't ordinarily pay much attention to. These wishes are at the periphery of your perceptions. Before you retire for the evening, reread these thoughts. Take them seriously. Start to see where these wishes might take you.

Don't go too far afield. Stay with the details you have written down during the day. This will help you find your way. Soon you'll carve out a direction that best suits you and your dreams. Once you trust your own voice and allow your creative force to come out, you will feel more fulfilled and more in touch with your feelings and subconscious. You previously did everything possible to avoid recognizing your deep dreams. Now you live them!

One of the most crucial things for you to do when you read this book is to listen to your own thoughts. Listening to yourself and to your environment lets you heal. Listen deeply. Think about your chronic pain. Listen and feel how you have reacted to it in the past and present. Listen with your whole body, not only with your ears, but with your hands, back of your neck and lower back.

Why designate a time to write? Because the timing helps pressure you to deal with your innermost feelings. You can better capture the moment of your feelings if there is a time constraint.

Putting feelings and thoughts on paper gives a concreteness to them, and creates a solid foundation from which to build. This is your opportunity to write down the obsessions, ideas, thoughts and feelings that haunt you. By expressing your obsessions in writing, you no longer need to displace them in the form of chronic pain. Your obsessions manifest a great deal of power over you, so it's best to recognize them in writing. Why allow them to take over your life and manifest themselves in your chronic pain? Why not get them to work for you?

When you express your feelings without any internal censor, your writing is energized, expressing the truth as you feel and see it. At first you may feel emotions and energy that will greatly concern you, and you may wish to stop your writing. Don't stop! Continue to record the details of your life, penetrating your most intimate feelings. Overcome your resistance.

Most of my patients resist the idea of writing their intimate feelings in a daily journal. But they soon realize how valuable writing is. Once they begin, many tell me, they wonder why it took so long to settle down and trust their deepest, innermost feelings.

When you write you go where your mind actually is, rather than where you think it should be. When you write what you first feel, your internal censor has no time to monitor what and how you feel. There is no time for "shoulds." There are no controls, so you can express what you truly feel.

Continue writing despite your pain. Persistence pays off; you'll gain confidence and control. This is the only way to attack the cause of your chronic pain. What could be better than to understand the emotion and feelings behind your pain? The benefits derived from writing are enormous.

Eric

No one was more surprised than I was when Eric, a construction engineer, successfully followed the steps in this exercise and chronicled his feelings and thoughts with great enthusiasm. Eric had been involved in a work-related accident. He had pain in his lower back and radiating down his left leg. The accident occurred five years before Eric entered my multi-disciplinary chronic pain center. Frustrated from unsuccessful treatments, Eric had resigned himself to days spent on the couch watching television. His family situation had deteriorated.

I warned Eric that he needed to get in touch with his feelings. I suggested relaxation, imaging, meditation, physical exercise and therapy. As an afterthought, I mentioned a daily journal to jot down his ideas, images, perceptions and feelings. By documenting his emotional and physical pain, I explained, he might uncover clues that would point him in new directions.

"I guess I'm afraid," Eric responded. "Afraid to allow myself to feel." But that's precisely what prevented Eric from going beyond his pain! Once he understood that putting pen to paper solidified his vague, ambiguous feelings, he began to reach his inner self. Writing helped Eric name the unmentionable by externalizing feelings with the magic of words. The abstract became concrete and tangible.

By keeping a daily journal you too can:

1. Release—not resist.

2. Face—not avoid

3. Explore—not hide.

4. Do. Change. Grow.

Creative visualization

Several times every day, my patient Michael mentally soars

above a beautiful beach like a bird. The stiffness and tightness in his upper back and neck dissolve, and he feels pain-free ecstasy. Michael uses the image of a bird soaring in the clouds as a metaphor to dissolve his pain.

In creative visualization you focus on your pain, then go beyond it. Lulled by a positive image, the conscious mind wanders away from its preoccupations. You enter a dream-like state and the unconscious surfaces. Sink deeper into this state and you experience the peace of the inner self. Try it.

Pinpoint the center of your pain. Visualize it slowly melting away. Imagine that as this spot shrinks you easily perform physical activities and exercises. Center on your breathing, counting down from 20 several times. Let go a little more with each exhaling breath, relaxing your head, neck, shoulders, arms and hands. Take more breaths, letting go with each exhaling breath. Do the same for your back, hips, thighs, knees, legs and feet. Let this sensation travel down your legs, right into the bottoms of your feet. As you see that pain spot become smaller and smaller, imagine that the range of motion throughout your body is more flexible. Now separate yourself from that pain spot by visualizing yourself floating on a cloud away from your body.

Try another visualization. See yourself floating on a raft, dumping your pain into the ocean while you simply float away. The power of imagination can turn what you visualize into reality.

Consider a very different kind of visualization, that of the Heisman football trophy winner. When running the ball, Charles White visualized himself as a bowling ball running through pins. During plays he also told himself he could vanish into thin air. He appeared to do exactly that when someone tried to block or tackle him.

"Mental reviews" of physical activities are known to cause muscle movements. The East Germans and Soviets use creative visualization as part of their athletic training. The more you can imagine an improved self-image or a body free of pain, the deeper your mindset becomes. The body cannot tell the difference between what is actually happening and what you have imagined or created. Like those athletes, you will have incorporated your visualization into your being.

The color is pain

For centuries, Eastern societies have mastered pain control. In researching their successful techniques, I found that the one common denominator in pain control is mental imagery. Even if you bring this concept into the sphere of scientific Western medicine, you can easily see its validity.

Dr. C. Norman Shealy, internationally known neurosurgeon and founder of the Pain and Rehabilitation Center in La Crosse, Wisconsin, taught a form of pain imagery to over a 1,000 chronic pain patients. Dr. Shealy claimed that pain imagery "is the number-one plan to stop pain. It is the single most effective therapeutic technique—bar none. It is more effective than drugs. And it works on headaches, backaches, arthritis and any other kind of pain."

Dr. Irving Oyle, professor at the University of California at Santa Cruz, confirms Dr. Shealy's findings through treatment on 1,000 patients of his own. He states, "Imagery is the most effective pain reliever I know. It really works on any kind of pain—from tension headaches to pain from muscles, joints and even from terminal cancer."

Dr. Dennis Jaffe of the Department of Psychiatry at UCLA Medical School reports that imagery becomes a way of communicating directly with your body. "You can achieve pain relief by using only the power of your mind—your imagination," according to Dr. Jaffe.

Exercise: To begin your first imagery exercise, choose a spot and time that afford absolute quiet. Distractions such as the telephone, a child yelling or a dog barking will interfere with the concentration necessary for successful imagery.

Sit in a comfortable position. Close your eyes and relax. Breathe deeply and slowly while you count down from 20. Drift into a deeper, more relaxed state with every exhaling breath. Imagine a color, and picture it as a sphere of bright light about six inches in diameter. Imagine it becoming larger and larger until it fills your field of vision. Now imagine it becoming smaller—shrinking—until it's only an inch or so in diameter. Finally, it disappears. Repeat this process, only this time imagine that the color is pain.

With a powerful image to control your pain, you create a force to which your mind and body can respond. Work diligently to create a fixed image you can call upon at will, and this image becomes a self-generated, specially coded message to combat your pain. With practice, controlling your chronic pain will become as spontaneous and automatic as controlling voluntary functions.

You will respond to imagery in one of two ways: in the abstract (utilizing subjective imagery) or in the concrete (using objective imagery).

If you can deal with the abstract, you can change your perception of pain by using symbols. You can creatively interpret your pain by using a symbolic expression—an image that clearly communicates how your pain feels to you. Almost a century ago, Carl Jung used symbols for dream interpretation and for unveiling subconscious and unconscious thoughts. You can apply his methods to symbolize and treat your pain.

Using symbols, you can tell your mind that the ultimate goal is to eliminate pain, and your internal system has an astonishing sense of what you're trying to communicate. Through imagery you can link your mind and body to "talk." You can use symbols to transform painful messages into pleasant perceptions. As long as you effectively communicate your needs, your mind and body will do what you ask.

Autogenic exercises are a more concrete method of getting similar results. Autogenic theory was developed in Germany during the late 1920s by Wolfgang Luthe, M.D., and Johannes Schultz, M.D. It consists of six standard formulas to suggest control of specific bodily functions. These formulas, as originally developed, are:

1. Heaviness

2. Warmth

3. Calm heartbeat

4. Regular breathing

5. Abdominal warmth

6. Cool forehead

When these are combined and the body responds positively, a homeostatic, or stable, condition is created in which you can control certain body functions.

To begin this autogenic exercise, assume a comfortable position, such as lying on your back on the floor. Close your eyes and wipe away tension with your imagination. Starting with one side of your body, imagine tension slipping away from your toes. Say to yourself, "My toes feel heavy. They feel heavier and heavier. My toes are sinking into the floor. Now my foot is getting heavy...," and so on, up one side of the body, then the other, until even your eyes feel relaxed. Now envision your entire body serenely floating away. Perform this exercise twice a day, preferably midday and evening.

If you cannot interpret your experience of pain using symbols or metaphors, try objective imagery. Objective imagery focuses on the physical site of your pain, and can create an image strong enough to let you experience what is happening within your body as it happens. For your specific perception of pain, you must develop a specific perception to counteract the pain.

Andrew

Andrew, unable to use subjective imagery, successfully alleviated his neck pain through objective imagery. Andrew's severe neck pain greatly restricted his range of motion. In fact, he was unable to move his neck. Yet he was unable to come up with a specific image of his neck pain.

But Andrew had read extensively about neck pain and attended various chronic pain lectures in his community on chronic pain. He was determined to take responsibility for his pain by doing everything feasible to understand his condition.

Although unable to experience his neck pain in terms of symbols or images, Andrew could identify the exact site of his pain and imagine the soft tissues in his neck strangulating and constricting the neck's nerves. In effect, this was Andrew's objective image. Next, he created a sense of release; that is, he was able to make the soft tissues release their hold on his nerves and allow energy to flow freely.

Hypnosis

A third form of distraction is the technique of hypnosis. The American Medical Association defines hypnosis as "a temporary condition of altered attention in the subject which may be induced by another person and in which a variety of phenomena may appear spontaneously or in response to verbal or other stimuli. These phenomena include alterations in consciousness and memory and increased susceptibility to suggestion. Further, phenomena such as anesthesia, paralysis, the rigidity of muscles, and vasomotor changes can be produced and removed in the hypnotic state."

In the hypnotic state, individuals learn to control pain in the same way they do with relaxation techniques. Learning to hypnotize yourself requires a great deal of responsibility and active involvement. You learn how to exert control of those biochemical reactions and electrical charges that occur in the complicated transmission of the pain signal from the pain site to the highest center of the brain. You learn to change the perception, the muscular response and the verbal and emotional reaction. The individual who has controlled his pain by hypnosis under the guidance of a physician has lost some of the fear of pain. With self-hypnosis you feel less and less like the helpless victim as you manage your pain sensation.The hypnotic state is a condition midway between being awake and being asleep. The hypnotized person can walk, talk and even write. In the hypnotic state, your conscious mind is "asleep." All suggestions are funneled to the subconscious mind. Hypnosis serves as a direct line of communication to parts of the brain, including the pituitary, which produces endorphins.

Endorphins are the key to controlling pain through hypnosis. It is hypothesized that hypnosis directs the brain to produce this painkiller. A person under hypnosis is very relaxed and highly suggestible. In this state, hypnotic suggestions for the reduction of pain seem to stimulate the production of endorphins.

You must undergo hypnosis under the guidance of a trained and certified professional. However, you can undertake a form of hypnosis on your own. Proceed carefully with this proven exercise. It may take several sessions to achieve deep relaxation, but the results are worth it.

1. Assume a comfortable position.

2. Take a deep breath and exhale slowly.

3. Close your eyes.

4. Lie back comfortably in the chair.

5. Let yourself go...loose, limp, slack.

6. Completely relax every muscle in your body.

7. Breathe in and out... slow and steady.

8. Stay with it until your entire body is loose and limber.

9. Envision each muscle getting heavier and heavier.

10. Once you become totally relaxed, you enter a state of semi-sleep. You are extremely quiet. Breathing becomes deeper and fuller.

11. In the deepest level of relaxation, your chronic pain subsides. You actually see endorphins filtering into every body part. As they permeate the skin and enter your body, your pain decreases.

Yoga and T'ai Chi Chuan

Yoga focuses on awareness, leading to natural transformation rather than forced change. No resistance is involved.

Transformation is the inevitable result of awareness; it is change that flows from a calm and tranquil center of identity.

Another approach is T'ai Chi Chuan, a traditional Chinese exercise that can work well with chronic pain individuals, especially those with joint stiffness, tenderness and swelling. It may also stimulate bone growth and strengthen connective tissues. T'ai Chi Chuan is the exact opposite of prolonged bedrest.

T'ai Chi Chuan combines deep diaphragmatic breathing and relaxation with slow and gentle movements. You gently stretch and increase the range of motion in your joints. You are encouraged to maintain good posture, as your movements flow imperceptibly from one into another. You will step with your full weight, but with a gentler heel-strike because you slowly and deliberately place your foot downward.

I am optimistic about T'ai Chi Chuan for individuals with chronic pain, especially chronic pelvic pain, because this very physical exercise is intimately linked to meditative exercises. Vital energy circulates throughout the body and systematically overcomes any blockage in the body's flow. For individuals with chronic pelvic pain, this exercise can relieve pelvic congestion and stoppage of bloodflow to the pelvis.

The graceful, meditative stretching movements of T'ai Chi limber the body, tone muscles and release tension. T'ai Chi employs a series of postures and hand movements linked like a string of words in a sentence. There are as many as 156 movements, depending on the form of T'ai Chi.

The self

Trying to describe the inner self in words is like trying to describe sweetness to someone who has never tasted sugar. You turn inward in meditation. Through deepening meditation, your unconscious takes form, reaches the surface and becomes visible. As you meditate and go within, you leave behind the external world of the senses. Albert Einstein, Charles Lindbergh and many others have made eloquent attempts, but the self still remains easier to experience than define.

Some call the self the "inner witness," the deepest part of the self, aware of all we think, feel and do. Even when we sleep, the inner witness knows whether we dream, and whether the dreams are "good" or "bad." The witness goes beyond the judgments of the mind and ego. Becoming aware of the witness or self in meditation, we experience an unconditional state. Our personal history, with all its fears, depression and pain, melts away. In its place comes a sense of oneness. For this reason, the self is often thought of as the unifying principle that links every human being to every other, and to the universe.

Coming home

Touching your inner self will raise your self-esteem and paint your outlook in brighter colors. It frees even the most negative individual from the pain/depression/insomnia cycle. You can separate from your pain. Your mind allows you to triumph over physical ailments.

Catherine

Catherine had a great deal of resistance to "new theories" to control her chronic pain. She was unsuccessful with all kinds of cures. But she never attempted to connect her chronic pelvic pain with the core of her inner self. Although Catherine was deeply religious, she needed to accept Jungian and Eastern philosophy to search within and transform her pain. Touching her newborn grandchild grounded her, and led to a belief in creative imaging, meditation and relaxation. This immediate connection provided Catherine with the sense of inner self she had been searching unsuccessfully for.

You do not need an experience like Catherine's to awaken you to that inner search. What is necessary is a sincere desire to transform your life and a willingness to open yourself to this new approach.

We may experience the self at any time, because the self is always within us. Usually the chattering of our minds keeps us from being aware. Anything that distracts us from our stream of negative, anxiety-producing thoughts allows us to experience the self. This is the purpose of meditation and deep breathing. In meditation we simply witness our thoughts. By detaching from old, outworn ways of thinking, we open to new and positive ways to deal with pain and life.

This is why meditation is like coming home. We find within ourselves the solace and security that we sought in vain from the outside.

*Those too eager to take pills are often the ones
trying to medicate their inner feelings.
They don't want to put up with any sort of discomfort.*

Goodbye to Drugs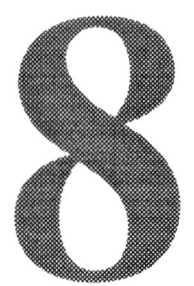

Searching on the outside for answers to pain that originates on the inside leads you on a downward spiral. The answers you come up with time and again are drugs and alcohol. Even pre-scribed drugs are trouble. Being addicted to Percodan, Xanax or Halcion is no different than being addicted to crack or alcohol. Because a doctor prescribes your pills doesn't make them good for you. You might not realize you are addicted. You make the reasonable but false assumption that because your doctor gave you the prescription, you can't possibly be addicted.

And what about those seemingly innocuous pills to quiet your nerves and allay your anxieties? They seem innocent enough, but are as addictive, habit-forming and dangerous as street drugs. You build a tolerance to them. Over time, more and more medication is needed to do the same job. Most medica-tions do nothing for chronic pain; they only dim concentration and awareness.

We are pill-obsessed. We are bombarded by pain killer adver-tisements on television, radio, magazines and newspapers. Why not? Fearing pain, we want to eliminate it from our lives, regard-less of the long-term consequences. Pills are a surefire answer.

Pills appropriate for an occasional headache or acute back strain have mind-numbing, debilitating side effects when used for chronic pain. Besides causing addiction, sedation, anxiety, sleep disturbance and even psychosis, they inhibit the release of the body's natural pain killers, the endorphins and enkephalins. The people too eager to take pills are often the people trying to medicate their inner feelings. They don't want any discomfort. But more pills over more time makes you more detached from your feelings.

If you are like my patient Sol and wash your pills down with whiskey and beer, you aggravate the problem. Or if you are like Allyson and combine pain killers, sleeping pills and tranquilizers, you are creating a life-threatening synergistic effect. Before Allyson entered the chronic pain control program, she was unaware of the danger of various drug combinations. Allyson thought more was better, and that eventually she would discover the right combination to make her pain go away.

Many drugs for chronic pain cause depression. Valium, a muscle relaxant, also produces depression. Narcotics like Percocet and Percodan alter mood as well as pain. They too bring sadness and depression.

The problem of addiction is greatly enhanced by drug combinations. Health care practitioners are increasingly aware of the role of drug dependency in perpetuating pain. Thus, for my patient Sol and countless others, providing a therapeutic environment for dealing with this dependency in crucial. Through a therapeutic environment someone like Sol regains control of himself and gets to know his inner feelings.

Sol

Sol thought nothing of mixing his tranquilizers, sleeping pills, addictive pain killers and beer. It had become natural for him—like taking a handful of vitamins! He was unaware that his drugs greatly contributed to his depression, anxiety, deteriorating interpersonal relationships and, yes, his increased pain.

By the time Sol entered the chronic pain multi-disciplinary center he was so detached from his feelings that he spent enormous energy restoring his sense of self. The combination of drugs and alcohol stripped him of his core identity.

Sol's turning point came when he realized, "I cannot take this any more." For Sol, step one was to admit and discuss his use of addictive medications. Simply making that statement to another person helped relieve a tremendous burden that Sol was carrying alone. Reaching out for someone is far better than reaching out for drugs.

Exercise:

1. Make a daily list of the drugs you take and note every time you take one. This makes your drug intake a reality.

2. Now do the same with your alcohol intake.

3. List those people with whom you can discuss your drug and alcohol intake. Select those with whom you feel comfortable and who are not too judgmental. You don't need a scolding. Talk with people who can be compassionate.

4. Discuss your medications with your doctor—even if you are sure you're not addicted. Tell your doctor all the drugs you are taking, including medications obtained through other physicians, dentists or friends. The problem of an original prescription being repeatedly refilled happens far too often in a busy medical practice. If your doctor doesn't respond to your satisfaction, find a doctor who will work with you to reduce your drug dependency. Or do it on your own. Take responsibility for your own health care.

My medication reduction program will not take away your drugs only to leave you with no alternative means of pain control. It will teach you to substitute drugs with relaxation training, creative visualization, imaging, meditation and all the tools needed to search within. This is combined with a physical exercise program to take you to your limit in range-of-motion exercises and conscious awareness of your body movement. Communication within your family replaces the oblivion and escape from thoughts and feelings associated with drugs. These techniques will help you cope with the nervousness and anxiety that made you turn to pills and alcohol.

Susan

For Susan, creative visualization and meditation addressed deep inner needs for self-love and spiritual fulfillment. She began to realize that her spiritual yearnings were being drowned by pain pills. Taking enough pills made Susan numb. The angst wasn't there, but neither was the joy. After she replaced pills with meditation and creative visualization, Susan was no longer fearful or detached from her feelings. She was now eager to deal with them. The age-old prescription for retraining her mind worked well for Susan. She learned to calm her mind and experience peacefulness and the contentment of her inner self.

Restoration of Susan's inner balance restored a part of her consciousness deadened by drugs. When Susan took responsibility for her pain and realized that she could not handle the drugs safely, she finally regained control over her life.

Bill

Bill refused any alternative to pain pills and tranquilizers. He saw only one way out: the television, a six-pack of beer and pills. Instead of substituting a more meaningful way of living, he continued his no-win lifestyle, all the while feeling helpless and hopeless.

Pills and alcohol entrenched Bill into a life of emptiness and spiritual dearth. He had become so detached from and unaware of his feelings that he sat in total oblivion. Bill refused to meditate and wouldn't acknowledge his drug and alcohol dependency. I was powerless to help him, so I encouraged Bill to seek psychotherapy.

Psychologists encourage people like Bill to examine the tension they may have denied and resisted for years. If you are addicted to prescribed medications and unable to use the methods in this book to get clean, you too may need a hospital or substance abuse treatment center to withdraw from drugs.

Establishing goals deserves high priority early in your recovery. You must establish specific well-activity behaviors and discourage chronic pain behaviors. But first, make it clear to yourself why you want to avoid certain activities. Ask:

•Why do I wish to improve?

•What would I like to be able to do?

Many individuals recognize that the amount of narcotic medication they consume is disproportionate to their pain. They increase the dosage to a point where they must devise elaborate schemes to account for a 30-day prescription consumed in two weeks. They may recognize imminent or existing addiction, but they are helpless to deal with it.

Keeping a medication diary

The medication diary is an expansion of the exercise suggested earlier in this chapter. It is a simple, inexpensive way to determine whether you are addicted to your medications. You and a family member should each keep a diary, recording the medications you take, when and how much. This crucial first step must not rely on memory. The process of documenting the drugs or alcohol you take for your pain or your anxiety is important. You can concretely see what you are taking, and this helps crystalize your problem. Seeing it on paper can convince you that there is indeed a problem. Are you mixing drugs innocently or intentionally?

When you document your drug intake, you begin to understand what drugs do to your mind, emotions and body. Yes, eliminating all drugs is a fearful prospect once you are conditioned to believe that pills are all that protect you from unbearable suffering. That's why taking this step alone might decrease your discomfort and increase your well-being.

Drug combinations can be lethal. If you are taking medications every three or four hours, there is a strong chance that you are addicted. Using drugs this way is actually a secondary gain for having pain. On a conscious level you tell yourself it's OK to take drugs to relieve pain. But you are telling your subconscious that it's OK to wash anxiety away with tranquilizers, sleeping pills and/or alcohol.

A medication diary also tells you how you feel when you do not take drugs. How anxious do you feel? Do you develop unwelcome withdrawal symptoms—nervousness, jitters, anxiety, sleeplessness, depression, increased perception of pain? Debra confided that when she tried to stay away from her drugs for a few extra hours, she would develop a terrible free-floating sense of anxiety and a fear that her pain would overwhelm her. Debra felt her world caving in on her, her breathing accelerating uncontrollably. Her hands trembled, she developed a bothersome twitch in her cheek, and her tongue bobbed in her mouth.

The fixed-time interval plan

While a detoxification program in a hospital may be necessary, the following procedure has been used to avoid increased demands for medication. Taking medications at fixed times rather than "as needed" averts the danger of pills becoming rewards for pain. This new pattern for taking medications guarantees a more stable blood level and allows you to decrease the pills you consume. Slowly, you can wean yourself from addicting medications and take control of your life. How? Rather than you trying to keep track of four or five medications, your pharmacist, under your physician's supervision, can combine your medications into a cherry elixir "Pain Cocktail."

The idea is to mix narcotic pain medication in a liquid-masking vehicle so the amount of narcotics you take can gradually be decreased. You are fully aware of the intended reduction, but you don't receive cues as to amount or timing. You take the cocktail at scheduled intervals, whether or not you are experiencing pain. Never do you take it between intervals, no matter how much you may want to or feel you need to. The average time interval is set at every four hours.

With your doctor's guidance, the pharmacist reduces the strength of your pain cocktail every week. It is a gradual but definite reduction until you no longer require any drugs. This method is far superior to a dramatic withdrawal, which can frighten and confuse you because of the symptoms it will produce. If you have used pain medication and anti-anxiety drugs over a prolonged time, there is a buildup of unmetabolized drug in your body. A sudden withdrawal wreaks havoc on your central nervous system and can cause seizures, disordered thinking, convulsions or unrelenting tremors. By gradually reducing your intake of pain cocktail, you safely eliminate your addiction to prescribed drugs.

Once the narcotic has been completely withdrawn from the liquid vehicle, a period which takes from four to eight weeks, you should discontinue the liquid.

Monitoring

Reducing your medication isn't easy. It requires constant monitoring. You can be your own medication monitor, but this places you alone, without outside support, and that is not what you want. Isolation is your enemy. Your goal is to drive yourself out of isolation and become part of society.

Alcoholics Anonymous, Weight Watchers and other support groups suggest that you pick a buddy: your spouse, a family member or a friend. Even better, connect with someone with a similar problem. The two of you can discuss your daily or even hourly frustrations and successes in controlling your drug intake. Your sense of connection with that other person becomes an invaluable reinforcement.

Knowing that someone out there cares about your success is a powerful incentive. Reach out to someone who will help you stick to your program and provide consistent and strong support as you gradually take control. Sharing innermost thoughts and feelings with this buddy will give you a new sense of release and freedom: You no longer have secrets. Discussing your addiction with a buddy gives it less power and control over you.

Pain support group

Another way to fortify yourself as you reduce your medica-tion is to organize a support group for chronic pain patients. Become involved. Be a motivator. Working on your own special project has far-reaching effects. Actively participating and giving your time will make you feel needed and productive. "Giving back" is one hallmark of self-help groups. When you give all that you have, focusing your energy, time, feelings, compassion and empathy on others, you are less preoccupied with your own troubles. Giving instead of taking (drugs) ignites your spirit and touches your soul.

Susan helped older individuals at the pain center who suffered from severe arthritis. Perhaps the most important thing Susan could do to avoid depression was to seek companionship and meaningful social interaction. She, like others with chronic pain, was a victim of isolation, spending much of her leisure time at home. By helping these older people increase their flexibility with various range-of-motion exercises and mobility training, Susan was less preoccupied with her own chronic pain. The satisfaction she received from helping others energized Susan to tackle her problem.

Individuals who communicate with others heal faster, feel less pain, are more motivated and less depressed than those who are isolated. Group members share words—and thus their worlds—by identifying with the troubling situations other group members discuss. In a group you can help each other identify troubling situations, ending your own self-absorption. You gain the confidence and insight to tackle your own problems without undue mental and emotional stress.

Building a social network

"I'm lonely."

"I have no friends."

"I don't know how to meet people."

You hear these statements from unhappy and depressed individuals with chronic pain. If you recognize yourself in these statements, this next exercise will help you.

You need a social network to help you stop wallowing in self-pity over your chronic pain. Complete isolation and self-absorption satisfy no one. A social network is your security base: You feel you belong. The group members know you and accept you. You realize what you can and cannot expect from each other. Whether you think of it as a support group or social network, the aim is clear: End self-absorption. Move on!

A social network includes all kinds of relationships—from superficial to very close. Your social network must suit your needs. The criterion for an adequate network depends not on the number of people but on the kinds of people and the variety of relationships available to you.

You can develop an assertive social network by seeking events—an office party or lecture, for example—where you might meet people you want to include in your social network. The best route to increased social activity is to follow your own interests. Participate in something you like and you are likely to be at your social best. Find an interest important to you and get active in it. By taking definite action you will get positive reinforcement. Eventually this will lower your anxiety.

If you still feel tense about new relationships, use reinforcing mental images to reduce the fear. Concentrate on the behavior you're afraid to perform—in this case, engaging in social relationships—rather than on your fear and concern.

Break the feared behavior into small parts, and use reinforcers. Anything that evokes a feeling of pleasure can be a reinforcer; it doesn't have to be connected with the act you are trying to reinforce. As long as the reinforcer gives you a good feeling, it will work. Once the reinforcing image is clear in your mind, say to yourself, "Reinforce" and immediately make the mental switch to the feared behavior. Do this exercise several times daily until you can perform the feared behavior in real situations with minimal anxiety. When you have the opportunity to engage in social relationships and form networks, perform the behavior step by step, as you did in your imagination. If necessary, switch to your reinforcing image to avoid anxiety.

Exercise: This self-revelation exercise helps you interact with people and form bonds in your chronic pain support group. You learn to tell very personal stories, which is important in pain support groups.

1. Take an important emotional experience from each decade of your life and tell them aloud, either to yourself or into a tape recorder. The stories can be happy, sad or trivial, but they must be events that had tremendous emotional significance for you.

2. Tell each story to someone with whom you want greater closeness—a spouse, close friend or an acquaintance you'd like to make into a friend.

3. The most important and difficult step? Tell your greatest trauma.

Revealing these stories starts you on the track of closeness and invites others to share their own meaningful experiences. It generates group closeness because it forces group members to deal with similar feelings and fears.

As closeness develops, pain support group members have greater behavioral flexibility. You share your feelings with greater directness and openness. You learn how to bring misunderstandings into the open and how to argue about personal issues. You share more because you know what to share.

Let's review your goals in a self-help group or social network:

1. Let yourself share and feel your feelings with others.

2. Feel free to communicate. It's OK to talk about problems. Be vulnerable. Feel free to need help and to ask for it.

3. Do what you need to do, what feels right. Don't just do the "right" thing.

4. Be who you are, without living up to another person's definition of you.

5. Communicate directly and clearly.

As group dynamics get more personal, fears of openness among group members vanish. In the group setting, do what you want to do and say what you want to say. Don't worry about whatever fear your actions generate among other group members.

Chronic pain support groups meet regularly, like Alcoholics Anonymous. You discuss common problems and further each other's growth and progress. Use the 12-step program as a model for your meetings.

During the first few weeks of your reduced medication program, the group should try to meet each day. This will be a constant reminder of your inner strength to cure yourselves. You are each rekindling your spirituality by surrendering to a strength and power beyond yourselves.

You each follow your own unique pattern, but together you produce a fabric of unity. Each of you will develop independently, but just as your emotional, spiritual, physical and mental components are interconnected, so too are the members of the group. All interdependently control each other's drug regimen. Group support multiplies exponentially.

Under the group's critical but supportive eye, you must willingly dissect your actions and thoughts, then help each other rearrange them into healthier ways of thinking and living. Being in touch with those who suffer similar difficulties reaffirms your commitment to stay off addictive drugs and shows how others struggle with similar circumstances.

Your support group must give its members plenty of reinforcement by stating affirming messages. This reminds the group of its deep concern and commitment to abandoning addicting drugs. Something like the following can be stated by each member during each meeting:

"I put my hand in yours and together we can do what we cannot do alone. No longer is there hopelessness. No longer must we depend on our own unsteady willpower. We are together, reaching out our hands for a power and strength greater than what any one of us can achieve individually. As we join hands we find love and understanding beyond our wildest dreams."

Affirmations

Affirmations are strong, positive, present tense statements. Affirmations make real that which you visualize. Your affirmations become your inner dialogue, thoughts that continually run through your mind. What you tell yourself—even if it might seem implausible—becomes the basis on which you experience reality. Affirmations change your negative mind chatter. Unhealthy attitudes that your pain has created are transformed into a positive reality.

Jim visualized himself doing physical exercises before he could actually perform them. However, the idea became entrenched in his mind. After many intense physical therapy sessions, he was physically ready to attempt his visualizations. And because he envisioned success, he completed the exercises and was ready for new visualizations of success.

Practice these seven affirmations. Then add a few that are uniquely your own.

1. I am in charge of my life and the path I choose.

2. My first priority is my own well-being and the journey of my soul.

3. I am responsible for my attitudes, feelings and behavior. I do not assume responsibility for the attitudes of others.

4. I am a fallible person who makes mistakes.

5. I learn from my mistakes and am accountable for them. As my behavior toward chronic pain becomes more appropriate, my success will grow.

6. I deserve to be treated with dignity.

7. There is plenty of time. I have the rest of my life to grow.

You are aware of how important it is for you to be an active participant in your support group. You have learned the skills necessary to be assertive within this group and to carry that confidence outside the group into other settings.

12-step approach to pain

12-step programs work very well. Most have one common theme: To help you connect with your soul and spirituality. The idea is to reach your inner self. 12-step programs replace emptiness with an uplifting sense of spirit.

The "thirst" of the alcoholic was seen by Carl Jung, who introduced the idea of spirit to the founders of Alcoholics

Anonymous. These founders believed that addiction is linked to lack of a connection to a higher principle. They realized that something equivalent to Jung's spiritual concept was necessary to conquer an addiction like alcoholism.

What Jung stated, and what any 12-step program encompasses, revolves around the search for the inner soul. Drugs and alcohol need to be replaced with a spirituality unique for you, whether or not you believe in a deity or supernatural being.

Meditation is one of the best ways to obtain spiritual growth. By meditating and cultivating inner silence, you achieve greater inner awareness. Inner awareness helps you avoid drugs and alcohol as escape mechanisms. Instead, you build confidence and willpower. With this expanded awareness comes recognition that your soul is separate from your physical body. This makes it possible to control that gnawing perception of pain. Inner silence strengthens healing and well-being. You have successfully substituted something external with something internal—something far more lasting and meaningful.

As this chapter began by stating, healing goes beyond your physical body when you turn to inner resources rather than the external to control pain. This inner connection makes it possible to retrain your mind to accept life, with all its problems, and rise above the pain that has enslaved you to drugs and alcohol.

*Effective pain treatment needs to occur within
your immediate environment,
and it needs to involve your family.*

Families in Pain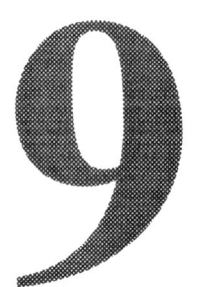

Theodore Roosevelt supposedly overcame severe asthma through vigorous exercise. But this claim partially skirts the truth. According to one biographer:

"Roosevelt had stopped suffering from asthma long before he took up the physical activities to which he later attributed his cure. The chief factor in his physical recovery seems to have been his removal from the family setting. When he went to Harvard his illness magically disappeared. The illness may have been psychosomatic. The only thing virtually all the attacks had in common was that they occurred on the same day of the week, Sunday: the one day of the week when Roosevelt's father was home and could take care of him."

Considering all that has been written about chronic pain, far too little has been said about the co-dependent family. When chronic pain occurs, it is symptomatic of pervasive problems. The dysfunctional family figures prominently in why someone develops pain and why the pain progresses from acute to chronic. As in any addiction, the entire family is properly "the patient," and the other members needs help and treatment as much as the person in pain.

Unless you are a hermit, your suffering is bound to affect your relationships, especially with close family members. In this chapter we explore the various roles that you, the chronic pain individual, play within the family unit, and how these roles, dele-terious to you all, are reinforced unconsciously by your family.

Books about chronic pain focus on the patient, usually dis-regarding the family. This book places great emphasis on your family. The family suffers considerably as a result of day-by-day problems caused by your pain. In the following pages we will explore the despair occurring within your family and the changes in family roles that often lead to extremely intense feelings of frustration, anger, guilt and apprehension.

Cures affected away from the home environment always seem to be fragile; as soon as the patient returns to the toxic set-ting where the pain originated, the pain problem recurs.

Claire

Claire, a New Jersey woman, lost 60 pounds while participating in a weight-loss program at Duke University. She and 40 other patients resided in a nearby hotel and participated in a rigid diet and exercise program at the hospital. During the three months she was there, her days were filled with planned hospital pro-grams; her evenings included group support sessions with the other patients and all kinds of activities. Claire seemed to make splendid progress. However, within a few months of coming home to an unhappy marriage—her husband was rarely at home, and when he was he basically ignored her—and an anxi-ety-provoking teenage son, Claire regained every pound she lost.

Why? She needed to fill her stomach with food to relieve the emptiness inside. She was a dieter who lost weight by placing herself in an environment far removed from her own. However, once back into the old environment, the eating began again, erasing all the progress she had made.

Effective pain treatment needs to occur within your immedi-ate environment, and it needs to involve your family. It has to have the continuity of care provided by a physical therapist, occupational therapist, psychologist or social worker in your community, not someone hundreds of miles away. Above all, it must address the interpersonal significance of pain. This means that every family member must acknowledge his or her role before the healing process can begin.

The ties that bind

Pain always affects family relationships and restructures family roles. Your pain evokes a wide range of feelings and behaviors in your family members. At first, your relatives may respond with concern and provide whatever comfort and help they can.

However, when the pain persists, feelings of anger and associated guilt may surface, especially when the pain causes inconvenience and difficulties for the family. Your spouse may have to deal with your depression, anxiety, loss of self-esteem, increased dependency, decreased sexual function and, in many cases, role reversal in employment. Your children may face emotional distancing due to your preoccupation with pain. They may experience the loss of an important role model. More upsetting, they may associate your illness with impending death.

Most individuals learn to express their chronic pain. You may find that when you complain of pain you receive a great deal of attention from your spouse. A marginally attentive husband, for example, suddenly becomes tenderly concerned when his wife expresses pain. After making sure she is comfortable and has plenty of medication, he prepares meals, washes the dishes, takes care of the children—all help she has pleaded for in the past. If she stops complaining of pain, he reverts to his usual inattentiveness. In this way the husband teaches his wife to express pain, because expressing pain produces secondary gains that would not occur otherwise.

Sympathetic friends and neighbors may act in the same way to influence expressions of pain. If the individual says he feels better, the visits from family, neighbors and friends often become less frequent. The individual with chronic pain quickly learns that to maintain social contact one must continue to express pain.

Expressing pain can help avoid an unpleasant situation. Pain offers a socially acceptable reason not to engage in certain activities. Society is more willing to accept a statement like "I can't because of my back pain" than "I don't want to."

It is not difficult to see how you might cling to pain behavior if it removes you from an unpleasant situation. Similarly, you may return to unhealthy habits rather than accept a new, pain-free lifestyle.

Doug

Doug, a 42-year-old oil field worker, had two unnecessary back surgeries and had become seriously addicted to medications before he was referred to me. He vehemently professed a desire to return to work and support his wife and teenage children, but refused all treatment other than surgery.

He also insisted that his wife not work, and she complied. Neither would face their situation and take purposeful action. They existed on Social Security disability payments. Doug and his wife chose the passive path, insisting they were victims of the "system." When I last saw Doug, he still insisted on more surgery, even though his previous surgeries had not helped his back pain and his surgeon had told him there was nothing left on which to operate. His wife, feeling helpless, had separated from Doug.

Your family's reaction to your pain may be anger, guilt or underlying doubt that your pain is real. This may cause them to react negatively or withdraw from you, and increase your sense of isolation. Conversely, they may be driven by guilt to give you far more help than you need. When family members encourage illness behavior and invalidism, it may indicate an unconscious desire to control or punish you, or a need to feel needed. Some people feel secure only when someone depends on them.

Faye

An example is Faye, the unmarried 50-year-old daughter of my patient Mildred, who suffered from rheumatoid and osteo-arthritis.

Faye welcomed walking her mother to my medical office, though they didn't live very far away. I called Faye the "Queen of the Waiting Room" because she clearly shined there. Faye took charge as soon as she and her mother walked in, offering other patients coffee and magazines and looking after their children. Sadly, as her mother's progress made her more independent, Faye became increasingly depressed and dysfunctional. She eventually fell sick herself, suffering from asthma and other pulmonary problems.

With an invalid in their care, people like Faye feel little likelihood of abandonment. They feel secure. Thus, both pain sufferers and their families may be locked into pathologic relationships that satisfy their symbiotic neuroses.

Do you use your chronic pain as an escape mechanism, a conscious or unconscious excuse not to do certain activities? This is how Jim used his chronic pain. Whenever he told his wife that his neck or back hurt, she said, "Oh honey, that's too bad. Why don't you go to the bedroom and rest? I'll take care of—" (whatever needed to be done). She would then admonish their children, "Don't bother your father right now. He is in a great deal of pain."

I have seen other individuals with chronic pain become manipulative to keep a spouse subservient or to regain the affection of a child or parent. The sufferer uses pain as the family theme, successfully solidifying all their supporting roles.

When I discuss the spouse's role in assisting his or her mate with chronic pain, I am discussing co-dependency. As one research team suggests, "The co-dependant is a spouse, child or other family member addicted to the person with alcohol, drug or other problems." Co-dependency is a way of relating to everyone and everything in life. It often involves deepseated unconscious needs for control and/or security.

Like the tendency to be pain-prone, the predisposition to co-dependency originates in dysfunctional families where parents were emotionally distant, tyrannical or abusive, or where emotions were repressed, falsified or denied. The quest for security drives the co-dependant to neglect his personal needs and become overly concerned with fulfilling the needs of those with whom he is intimately involved.

The husband of one of my chronic pain patients expressed it perfectly after recovering from a long and severe case of the flu. "Mary took care of me!" he confided with amazement. After 30 years of taking care of Mary, he could hardly comprehend this new experience.

Pain's history

Throughout childhood you learn to associate pain with two interactions: receiving help and care, or being punished. The degree to which pain plays a role in gaining care and attention during your childhood greatly influences the extent to which pain later becomes a coping strategy. You may come to communicate any form of distress, whether anxiety or depression, through various pain statements. Relief may not even depend upon other people's responses. Just stirring up memories associating caring with pain may encourage you to stop worrying about other people and lavish care on yourself.

Care and affection are given only following pain in some families, such as after a child has been physically punished or abused. The child soon believes that he or she is bad, lovable only after his or her imagined sins are punished.

These individuals choose the symptom of chronic pain to offset long-standing guilt. After years of clinical experience, psychiatrist George Engel reported that guilt is almost always a factor in choosing chronic pain as a symptom. It is rarely possible to experience pain and guilt simultaneously. It seems that a measure of guilt is neutralized by a measure of pain.

Engel's "pain-prone patient" was characterized as guilt-ridden, depressed and possessed of low self-esteem. Obviously, this broad generalization might not apply to you. For Engel's patients, it fit often enough to become the norm. His patients showed similar histories of punitive, abusive parents, with pain linked to early suffering and later used as an important form of communication.

Engel's patients could not deal with life's difficulties, and chose to be fearful rather than overcome fear. We all have fears; we must learn to overcome them and direct our lives as we desire.

Engel's female patients frequently had mothers who were chronically ill and in pain throughout their daughters' childhoods. In some cases the pain was attributed to the daughter's birth. The potential for guilt is obvious. Not surprisingly, these patients unconciously tended toward pain-producing situations, including unnecessary surgeries.

Perhaps you had your first attack of pain during adolescence. Thereafter, your attacks might have occurred when your need to suffer was not satisfied by external events. Many say their pain started "just as everything began to go well for the first time." Sometimes pain occurs as a response to a real or threatened loss of a significant person or possession. The pain may, in fact, symbolize the lost person and even parallel the pain suffered by that person. In this sense, pain allows the sufferer to expiate guilt toward the absent or deceased person. Pain helps attain psychological equilibrium, especially when the sufferer feels guilt.

Guilt is a part of any pain problem. When you experience constant discomfort, your family, friends and co-workers are affected. A co-worker might have to assume your work load. Your spouse may have to supplement the family income. A child might forfeit a new bike because the money went to medical bills. Guilt is everywhere!

Take an active role

Communicating with family members will help you heal your chronic pain. When you discuss issues within the family, you create a greater closeness and have less need to use your pain to manipulate your family. Here are some steps to help bring about closeness.

1. Define your goal: To do anything that fosters direct, honest communication and diminishes the need to use pain to manipulate.

2. Write out what you want to say to each family member. Record it on a tape recorder. Review your words, concentrating on the "how." Make sure you talk about what is really on your mind.

3. Play back your message and make any necessary "script" changes. Check your emotional communication, your volume. Practice the message until it feels right to you.

4. Set a time to discuss these issues. Choose an hour when all family members are present and not too tired to discuss your pain. Make sure you get the message across. Sometimes you send one message while family members hear another.

Improve the way you make decisions in your home concerning household responsibilities, vocational activities, communication, personal independence, financial management and any other tough areas.

If you feel you make too many decisions, this becomes a burden that you resent, not a shared bond. Or you may resent other family members who control the decision-making. Communication helps you tally the number and kinds of decisions you make and those you would like to make. It can also help you decide what changes can be made and which areas are most important. Ask yourself these two questions:

1. How many of the decisions do I make now?

2. How many would I like to make?

Select one area you feel needs the most change. Discuss with each member of the family what you can do to create change in that area. Begin with the area in which you have the greatest chance of success. As you progress, move on to the next most likely area. Start with small steps and do one specific area at a time. Don't try to do too much at once.

The following guidelines create healthier family communication:

1. Talk to your family about how you feel. Be honest and open about your emotions and ask them to fully express their feelings.

2. With all family members present, list the responsibilities you can now accomplish. This redefines your role within the family.

3. Make it clear to all family members that everyone's roles change throughout life, and that your role will change as your pain vanishes.

4. Hold weekly meetings, at a designated time and day, to review family events over the past week. This forces better communication among family members. Good communication is the best weapon to combat guilt.

Re-enacting history

Your pain can serve a host of purposes within your family. Communicating pain, verbally or with body language, directs attention toward yourself and away from other matters. Your pain puts you in control. It may serve to gratify your need to be dependent and cared for, but your dependency may be quite a burden to your family. At the same time, you may unconsciously be punishing your family by being so preoccupied with pain.

Mrs. Siroti

A case in point is Mrs. Siroti. Outwardly sweet and compliant, Mrs. Siroti would only come for treatments for chronic back pain when her husband could accompany her. She was in her early forties and lived only blocks from the pain management center, but nothing could induce her to walk, drive or take a bus or cab. Chronic pain satisfied her strong dependent needs and hidden desire to control, while allowing her to avoid her marital problems.

Chronic pain is often a way of avoiding tasks, strained marriages, sexual problems or other commitments. By conferring the privileges of the sick, it permits irritability or rudeness without disapproval.

Invariably, chronic pain expresses deep inner turmoil that you are unwilling or unable to confront directly. In **Minding the Body, Mending the Mind**, Dr. Joan Borysenko cites the case of a man who became despondent when his pain almost disappeared. "Now I don't know what to do with myself," he said. "I'm 27 and I've never moved out of my parents' house. I don't know how to relate to women. I should probably go back to school, but I'm too scared. I don't know how to live any other way. I think I want my pain back."

Perhaps you, too, fear giving up pain, maybe with the covert support of your family. Your response to the questionnaire in Chapter 4 should give you an idea of the roles pain plays in your life. Recognizing those roles that do not foster well-being is the first step toward changing them.

Making a toxic environment healthy

Family can either boost your efforts to control pain or unwittingly sabotage them. In either case, it is in everyone's best interests for the people you live with to read this book and participate in your treatment program. Once you and your family understand what perpetuates your pain, you can work together to make changes.

The workplace is an important part of your environment, so what I have said about the family applies to co-workers as well. Patients constantly report increased pain due to stressful working conditions or fear of job loss. Stress management techniques such as relaxation training, biofeedback or hypnosis will help you minimize work-related stress and anxiety that contribute to your pain. Finally, the more you inform people at work about your efforts to control your pain and resume your normal functions, the more likely they will be helpful and supportive.

Family dialogues

Awareness of how we act helps us act how we want. An excellent way to examine how your persistent pain affects family members is for everyone to participate in a structured dialogue. Be direct with your communication. Say what you mean. The goal is for each person to become aware of his or her role in managing pain. Once aware of how you respond to one another, you can unlearn the habits that reinforce pain and substitute ones that strengthen well behavior.

Additionally, practice expressing emotions with someone you trust. Begin slowly. If that person offends you, explain how you feel and how his actions precipitated your feeling. Gradually you can explore how present feelings are tied to your past. Unleashing repressed feelings into current emotions helps to relieve internal pressure. Some of your reasons for holding your pain will then vanish.

If your problems and behavior patterns are deeply ingrained, seek the help of a psychologist or social worker trained in family therapy. Or consider a brief community education course on enhancing communication skills, often available through a mental health center.

Family and/or marital counseling builds communication. Family therapy teaches family members how to discourage pain behavior and help the sufferer regain independence and self-confidence. Therapy teaches family members to accept and respect their own natural resentments for assuming the burdens of the chronic pain individual. It helps them explore the unconscious messages they send.

For example, what does a spouse gain from a helpless mate? Freedom from sexual demands? Family control? Elimination of healthy competition? How can a spouse find more constructive, less painful ways to satisfy his or her needs and reach personal goals? Family therapy helps the spouse understand his or her own role in the pain syndrome and change behavior that rewards fear, helplessness and dependency in favor of behavior that encourages both partners to take charge of their lives and their responsibilities.

All in the family

Studies prove that psycho-social and family-related factors account for much of the variance in pain intensity and its interference in daily activities. By keeping pain diaries you, your spouse and other family members (or a program buddy) will connect heightened pain to specific events or behaviors. Each of you should note diligently each incidence of pain and what interactions or happenings preceded it. Note, too, those times when pain noticeably lessened, and what happened shortly before.

Medical studies have asked spouses to maintain a pain diary of their spouses' expressions of pain, time of day, location and their own feelings and perceptions. The conclusion? If they were solicitous toward the pain, the pain increased and the sufferer's activity level decreased, implying impairment in functioning. These studies demonstrate how important it is to include spouses in the treatment of chronic pain.

Your mate can learn to reinforce your well behavior and ignore your pain behavior. Family members can learn not to gang up on the patient, too. This is not an exercise of blame, but a plan for healing in which all family members work together to lessen one member's chronic pain.

Since the entire family is the patient, each family member should participate in relaxation and breathing techniques, creative visualization and meditation. Having each family member capture his or her inner self benefits the entire family.

Family support groups

Support groups such as Al-Anon and CODA (Co-Dependents Anonymous) are invaluable to families of those addicted to alcohol and drugs. There is no less need for a group for the families of chronic pain patients. I have instituted such groups in several of my pain management centers and found them immensely successful in helping families express their fears, anxieties, frustrations and anger.

Without question, living with a chronic pain patient stirs a variety of emotions. Family support groups attempt to rechannel those emotions into more positive feelings. They offer a place to discuss common problems, express pent-up feelings, receive care and understanding, and learn to cope. Ideally, they are led by trained facilitators, but they can be effective as weekly gatherings of friends or sympathetic people with similar problems.

If there is no existing group in your community, start one. All you need is a few interested people. The group should focus on the family and not on magical cures or omnipotent figures of authority. Placing matters on the family rather than depending upon large institutions reinforces the importance of the small but crucial family support system.

Design your weekly meetings as 12-step programs, emphasizing the practical and the inspirational. Strength comes from a higher power, which members can interpret as God, their inner selves, or whatever is most meaningful for them.

Dysfunctional family situations foster chronic pain and co-dependency. By contrast, healthy families acknowledge their problems and feelings openly. Each individual is encouraged to be independent, take chances, pursue individual pleasures and enjoy individual successes. Self-esteem comes from within, for reasons that are real, not from the opinions or achievements of others.

Each of us wants to be healthy, loving and self-confident. Chronic pain, paradoxically, can be your doorway to health in the broadest sense. It requires you and your family to accept pain as a challenge and a vehicle for growth. It happens by taking small, deliberate steps. If you continue, nothing can stop you from reaching your pain-free destination.

Your mind and body interface with one another like a couple of Olympic skaters.

From Childhood Abuse to Chronic Pain

10

Physical or sexual abuse in childhood or adolescence can surface as lower back or pelvic pain. One study shows that two out of three patients with chronic pelvic pain have a history of sexual abuse. In another study, 40 percent of chronic pelvic pain patients had been subjected to incestuous relationships. Women with chronic pelvic pain have a much higher incidence of sexual abuse than any other group.

At least one in four women are survivors of childhood sexual abuse. These women rarely reveal their history to their physicians. Many have never discussed the abuse with anyone. Over 60 percent of the victimized women felt they would have great difficulty discussing their experience with a medical professional or could not discuss it at all.

An integrated approach toward chronic pelvic pain lets the patient and those who treat her take into account previous sexual abuse. This is significantly more effective than the standard surgical treatment (laparoscopy) for chronic pelvic pain. Because unresolved continuing pain is unacceptable to both patient and physician, the decision to operate is made frequently and impatiently. The alternative to surgery is the multi-disciplinary approach. Because they emphasize holistic medicine, multi-disciplinary centers blend physical and psychological therapies.

Women treated for chronic pelvic pain at the gynecology clinic at Leiden University Medical Center in suburban Amsterdam are encouraged to partake in an integrated approach by working with a "psychosomatic physical therapist." They are also encouraged to make changes in their lives by working with the team's social worker. However, the majority of these women are unwilling to see the link between past abuse and chronic pelvic pain.

Nevertheless, the psychosomatic physical therapist encourages breathing, relaxation and postural exercises. If a patient resists, she is encouraged to talk with a social worker or physical therapist who is sensitive to sex abuse issues.

Below is a comparison of the multi-disciplinary approach toward chronic pelvic pain to the standard approach of laparoscopy.

	Laparoscopy	Integrated Approach
Total women	49	57
General pain experience		
Improvement	20 (41%)	43 (75%)
No improvement	29 (59%)	14 (25%)

	Laparoscopy	*Integrated Approach*
Interruption of activities		
Improvement	18 (37%)	39 (68%)
No Improvement	31 (63%)	18 (32%)
Associated Symptoms		
More	26 (53%)	4 (7%)
Some	10 (20%)	10 (18%)
Fewer	13 (27%)	43 (75%)

A woman with chronic pelvic pain has statistically more depression, learned helplessness, lifetime substance abuse, adult sexual dysfunction and other psychosomatic complaints, such as gastrointestinal difficulties. She is more likely to have had one or more major depressive episodes linked to learned helplessness.

By the time she seeks treatment, her chronic anxiety and related problems have become tools to cope with her fear of another assault or punishment by her aggressor/parent. She has little insight into her feelings of being trapped or victimized in her marriage, job or other interpersonal relationships. She may be unaware that suicidal thoughts and actions reflect her sense of helplessness. Like other pain sufferers, she cannot put her pain into perspective. It is merely a continuation of the negative experiences life hands her and for which she is somehow responsible.

A woman with chronic pelvic pain lives her life in shadows.

The past is a shadow. The future is shadowed by the past. Her relationships are shadows of previous relationships. When she interacts, she relives veiled reflections of past issues she has not resolved. In response to her pain, she allows herself to be herded by illusions of danger into little compartments of fear. She becomes a prisoner of shadows.

Women who are physically or sexually abused find their abuse difficult to deal with emotionally, so they block out their memories. By doing so, they contain their anguish and develop a sense of powerlessness. The shadow then gains great power. Rather than recognize it for what it is—a reappearance of past experiences—a large percentage of the abused use somatization: They convert their experiences, feelings and mindsets into physical symptoms. Fear, guilt, learned helplessness, powerlessness and internalized anger all lead to further physical deterioration.

Your mind and your body interface like a couple of Olympic skaters. Any physically and/or sexually abused woman has traumatic memories and pain trapped inside her. Unhealed and unresolved wounds result in feelings of alienation from herself and others. No wonder she has difficulty managing her chronic pain.

Several studies demonstrate that for abused women, somatization and denial are the primary coping styles. These women have more gynecological, gastrointestinal, neurological and musculoskeletal problems.

One early and important study on the link between sexual/physical abuse and chronic pelvic pain was conducted by Dr. G.M. Guzinski at the University of Washington Medical Center. Not one of the 100 women studied was found to have correctable pelvic pathology. However, 95 percent showed significant psychological pathology. Their histories revealed a prevalence of sexual abuse: 65 percent had been the victims of incest, rape or sexual molestation; 40 percent had been subjected to an incestuous relationship, usually with a stepfather or stepbrother.

Chapter 9 discussed family systems and their role in chronic pain. Women with chronic pelvic pain can also gain much-needed support from understanding family dynamics. What occurs within the family has far-reaching consequences for years to follow, embedding memories into the unconscious and subconscious.

Laura

Laura was both physically and sexually abused during her childhood and adolescence. Whenever she misbehaved or acted in ways her parents could not control, her mother and father would verbally and physically abuse her. As an adolescent, Laura was sexually abused by an older brother and her uncle. These abuses were never discussed among family members, and Laura learned not to acknowledge the abuse, even to herself. Instead, she repressed extremely painful and hurtful feelings in order to function.

As a young adult, Laura got a job, married and had two children. To survive, she pushed those hurtful feelings still deeper, dissociating those earlier events from her present life. In several ways Laura became a robot, devoid of feelings or emotions. However, during this same period she developed anxiety, depression and pelvic pain.

A shamed person lives with a sense of her fatal flaws and unrelieved worthlessness. Laura allowed her pain to intensify, and was overwhelmed by a sense of worthlessness. She believed giving up her pain would make her feel insecure and at a loss.

Laura had difficulty forming a close relationship with her husband because she felt inadequate about her femininity. She never acted directly with her husband; instead, she controlled their relationship with her chronic pain. She was uncomfortable confronting her husband when she was angry at him, but unable to recognize or express her discomfort. Instead, she accused him of being insensitive and ignoring her feelings.

Laura required a great deal of support from her husband in times of stress, yet he could never understand her complex emotional reactions. He could not be supportive because he could not understand why she reacted the way she did.

Laura entered the multi-disciplinary chronic pain program as a 45-year-old housewife with a long history of chronic pelvic pain. Together, Laura and I uncovered how her difficulty in externalizing her stress and hostility was directly related to her fear of severe retribution from her previous abusers. Her suppressed feelings led to the simmering inner turmoil that produced her chronic pelvic pain. Laura had frequent flashbacks, reliving the traumatic experience as if it were happening. From those flashbacks she learned about her initial trauma.

Slowly, Laura made progress. Using her inner guide through creative visualization and imagery exercises, Laura left her consciousness and returned to the flashback, gently re-experiencing the feelings and body sensations that it produced within her. The memories from the traumatic experience produced intense feelings and sensations.

Through deep-breathing exercises, she focused on her body and transcended the abusive experience. Her pelvic and lower back muscles relaxed. Her panicky feeling decreased as she felt less trapped within her own body. New feelings opened up for her, and Laura felt more connected with her body. Stuffed feelings and guarded, blocked memories were released. Laura freed herself of negativity as she worked through her feelings.

Every day Laura concentrated on her message: "I cannot ignore my pain, nor can I manage it alone. I recognize my feelings. I perceive the connection between my abuse and my behavior today. Breathing deeply, I imagine controlling that connection. I have a new sense of myself. I am in touch with my anger, yet I can detach myself from that anger. I have replaced it with a 'new' me, one filled with creative energy and newly found growth."

The focus of her therapy centered on Laura's ability to bring up repressed emotions. Her three goals were clear:

1. To identify her feelings.

2. To identify repressed emotions from her childhood trauma.

3. To bring into the open and address those feelings and repressed emotions.

Laura needed to become aware of her emotional life, not isolate herself from herself and others. This she accomplished by meditating and practicing progressive muscle relaxation, deep-breathing exercises, imagery exercises and creative visualization. Laura performed these exercises to remember the trauma. To heal, Laura needed to remember. With great detail, we worked with Laura to reconstruct what happened. We developed a tailormade program using techniques like writing, drawing, storytelling, cues, hypnosis and flooding.

Writing, drawing and storytelling about her initial and subsequent sexual and physical abuse helped Laura crystalize her feelings. In her own way she recorded her past. We identified and collected any objects, or "cues," that helped trigger her memory. After initial instruction, Laura performed these techniques herself. She was most skillful at reviving what occurred in her dreams, bringing feelings and emotions into her wakefulness and, thus, into her consciousness. This leaking-out process requires writing down your dreams and expanding on them utilizing some of Carl Jung's techniques.

Laura learned to forgive first herself and then those from her past. She learned how sensory and image flashbacks can uncover past events. Smells, colors and specific visual images became important in uncovering the traumatic experiences. It was difficult yet necessary for Laura to relive her intense feelings and body sensations.

Exercise:

1. Find a quiet, undisturbed place.

2. Take deep, long breaths.

3. State aloud that you are not upset for the reasons you think.

4. Focus on something that is a reminder from your unhealed past.

5. Forgive. Heal. Release.

Perform this exercise whatever your trauma is. After you find that quiet place, breathe deeply. Don't be distracted from this important focus and imaging process. Touch upon any image that might help you remember the trauma. As you delve into the trauma, discover its every component. Give it form, shape, smell. Give it a feel. As you proceed, you will discover that with healing comes forgiveness. You will forgive yourself and move on.

Hypnosis and flooding require strict supervision from psychologists at the multi-disciplinary center. Hypnosis brings forth repressed memories by creating a semiconscious state of deep relaxation. Flooding—or implosive therapy—has been used successfully with individuals who have been sexually/physically abused. I explain this therapy here, but please do not attempt it on your own.

In the treatment center, Laura was barraged with cues to remind her of her abuse. She reacted in whatever way was natural for her. Immediately following the painful memories were deep-breathing exercises and progressive relaxation. Alternating excessive, painful stimulation with calming relaxation served two purposes:

1. Re-creating the experience followed by serenity, centering and ultimately self-forgiveness allowed Laura to feel the trauma

on a deep, gut-wrenching level. She experienced guilt, anger, fear and grief. She re-experienced the self-blame she felt during the original abuse. She experienced the helplessness involved in traumatic episodes. But from these experiences she grew.

2. After getting in touch with her grief, Laura could move on. Her unresolved grief only worsened her pain. It caused her considerable anger, restlessness, rage, depression and conflict.

At the multi-disciplinary center, Laura learned acceptance and a new way of life. She stopped fighting her past. She learned how to support herself emotionally, making her life as meaningful as possible. After all, why should she allow her past to destroy her present and future? Laura turned trauma into empowerment. By centering herself, Laura could appreciate her emotional and spiritual growth. She took control over her life by accepting the emotional effects and perceived trauma scars. Using her new knowledge, Laura could now focus on her marriage.

Laura and her husband received assertiveness training. As a result, Laura no longer played the victim. In therapy with her husband, she shared the secret of her victimization and how the abuse affected her marriage. Trust increased between the couple. As Laura gained more control over her life—and over her pain—she felt less trapped in her marriage.

Laura realized she had a choice in every situation. When she played the victim, she was refusing to take responsibility for her situation. Once Laura realized that she had alternatives and could make choices, her feelings about her chronic pain changed.

It is difficult for those with chronic pelvic pain to reveal feelings about previous physical and/or sexual abuse to family members. It is equally difficult for them to disclose the abuse to their physicians. These women generally prefer silence. The failure of our legal system and our society leaves victims little choice but to hide and try to forget the experience. Victims may be beaten or threatened with further physical or sexual abuse if they resist. Frequently I hear, "I wasn't going to be heard, so I clenched my teeth and got through it." Faced with exile from the family, the individual learns to disown her feelings. But the experience lingers in her subconscious and unconscious, and translates into physical pain.

The humiliation never goes away. Because abuse remains hidden, unanswered and unchallenged, the very body, the physical self, becomes the shame. The "damaged" self reinforces the concept within a woman that she has lost power over her body. These experiences encourage a woman like Laura to allow chronic pain to control her. The ultimate betrayal has occurred: the betrayal of herself by her body. Because of past violations, she can no longer depend on what her senses tell her about her inner world or outer environment.

A victim suffers an omnipresent bleakness. No longer is it the specific abuse that weighs heavily, it is the thoughts and general aura surrounding the event. That is why it is so easy for the victim to believe, subconsciously or unconsciously, that chronic pain is a just reward.

Contrary to popular belief, forgiving helps the victim, not her abuser. If she does not forgive, she, not the abuser, remains chained to the events of the trauma. For it is she who is locked up with her fears and judgments. When she forgives, she is free of hurtful feelings and thoughts. I call this "daring to forgive."

I do not imply that one moment of forgiveness can erase a lifetime of fear and self-imposed guilt. Rather, the act of forgiving herself and her abuser releases energies previously consumed by anger, negativity and separation from her inner self.

Do not underestimate the power of forgiveness. Forgiveness provides the light in which all of your past, no matter how dark, is transformed into a new ability to seek and search. By forgiving past abuse, you gain freedom and healing.

Exercise: Think through these questions, then record your answers in your notebook.

1. List three misdeeds committed against you for which you still punish yourself.

2. List three past abuses for which you still think yourself the victim.

3. List every grudge and resentment you carry. Next to each, record the length of time you have been carrying it.

4. Are you willing to release some or all of these grudges? If so, write a statement of forgiveness next to the misdeed(s) you are willing to release.

5. What steps can you take to finalize this release? Write down what you might tell the individual(s) you want to release or forgive.

The most direct way to stop past abuse from continuing to damage your psyche is to remove your permission. Unresolved abuse issues permit that past episode to hold power over you.

No one needs to put up with abuse of any kind. That includes the self-abuse you inflict by clinging to past abuse. No one, including you, can hurt you unless you permit it. Not until you are willing to resolve your past abuse and put it to rest will you truly heal.

Regaining self-respect is pivotal to the healing of abuse. As you accept yourself and gain self-respect, you do not need others to validate your worth. You know you are important. Who else agrees is unimportant. Self-esteem is not founded on the approval of others; it comes from within.

Exercise: How can you transform situations to honor yourself more? Four questions to ask yourself:

1. When in your life do you feel disrespected?

2. Do you see patterns of abuse or disrespect?

3. Do you permit these situations to continue?

4. Do these situations reflect ways in which you do not respect yourself?

There is no reason for you to stay in a situation—emotional, spiritual or physical—that causes you damage. Yet most individuals resist change at any cost. Change is scary. It means dealing with the unknown. It entails utilizing inner resources and challenging inner dimensions. Yet the outcome can be marvelous.

It is quite likely that your sense of guilt, unworthiness and lack of self-esteem leads you to believe you must endure pain. You may also believe that you must continue to suffer to "pay off" previous trauma and abuse. I urge you to reclaim your right to pain-free happiness now! Treat yourself with dignity and respect, and watch it happen!

*Set a goal and you'll be pleasantly surprised
how often you reach it.*

Reconditioning Your Body 11

If you have been following conventional medical treatment for chronic pain, chances are you are in poor physical shape. For example, resting in bed, even for a couple of days, weakens your muscles. Become inactive for weeks or months and your muscles atrophy. More than 80 percent of chronic neuromuscular pain cases are caused by lack of exercise. Muscles that are weak, tense, rigid and inflexible are susceptible to numerous trigger-point pains.

With chronic tension, stress or pain, your muscles contract. This limits the blood that flows into that muscle, and with it a relaxing supply of oxygen. Tensed muscles also release minute amounts of "kinins," the pain-signaling by-products of muscle contraction. Kinins are warning messengers that act directly on the spinal nerves that transmit pain. When the muscle is in prolonged contraction, kinins signal the body to initiate relaxation. This allows an increased flow of blood and more oxygen to carry away the kinins. This is why individuals who suffer from tension and stress caused by chronic pain experience increasing discomfort by not exercising. Research shows that the more patients exercise, the less pain they have.

The story of football running back Rocky Bleier is convincing. After receiving severe wounds to a foot and leg in Vietnam, Bleier rejected pain and the predictions of his retirement from football. Instead, he redoubled his pre-war exercise program. In time, reporters noticed his superior strength and speed. "Pretty soon," he recalls, "an aura surrounded me. The coaches were touched by it. They heard the talk and read the papers like everybody else. Finally they said, "Hey, this guy is quicker and stronger. We gotta play him more."

An individualized physical therapy and exercise program may not prepare you for pro ball, but it can make you stronger, more flexible and more independent. My patient Mildred is a good example. Mildred had crippling rheumatoid arthritis. At the multi-disciplinary center she learned range-of-motion and stretching exercises. In short order, Mildred could walk on her own again and perform simple tasks without her daughter's assistance. The pain in her joints dramatically decreased.

The secret is to exercise toward your goal, not to do as much as you can or continue until it hurts. Set a goal and you'll be pleasantly surprised how often you reach it. But first, a caution: Before exercise, consider your medical constraints and limitations. Every individual with chronic pain needs a medical evaluation to prepare his physical exercise program. Individuals progress at different exercise rates. It is wise to ask a physical or occupational therapist to help you pace yourself.

In my medical practice I see many couch-potato patients who get no physical exercise. They are convinced that exercise will increase their pain and that rest is their answer. They couldn't be more incorrect.

Alan

When I first saw Alan he was 30 pounds overweight and complained of chronic, gnawing lower back pain. He did no exercises and ingested pain pills and sleeping pills that made him lethargic and inactive. Alan was surprised to hear that his sedentary lifestyle weakened his muscles, impaired his coordination, caused joint contractures and limited his motion. His lower back pain was hindered, not helped, by his inactivity. His weak abdominal muscles, and an extra 30 pounds of fat, produced further strain and stress on his back.

Alan enjoyed swimming as an adolescent, so he was encouraged to swim again, using various water exercises. The buoyancy of water allowed him to stretch his joints without stress. Alan also learned to walk briskly again, with particular attention to his posture so that pressure was not placed on his lower back muscles.

Become aware of your power

Walking allows the joints of your body to move freely without undue pressure on tendons, muscles and joints. Walking is something anyone can do in any situation. Walking improves oxygen consumption during exertion, lowers heart rate while resting, relieves accumulated psychological stress, increases muscle tone, reduces blood pressure, releases muscular tension (reducing pain) and increases heart and lung efficiency.

When you walk, stride comfortably. Begin with short walks to build endurance, but increase time and distance. Don't focus on speed. Take your time and move at a comfortable pace. Relax while you walk. Continuously check for tension build-up, especially in your neck and shoulder muscles.

Exercise:

1. Choose a route for a 20-minute walk.

2. Walk the route at least once a day. Be aware of your posture and how you carry your spine.

3. Keep your back straight, not hunched. Swing your arms

forward and back briskly. This provides movement and range for your upper body.

In the vast majority of pain cases, one underlying cause is an easily corrected problem: lower back pain often improves considerably if you simply lose weight.

By knowing your body, how it moves and how it works, you know your power to make yourself feel better. By exercising, you develop an entirely new lifestyle. What an empowering idea! Make your body strong and healthy. Take a walk. Breathe in the fresh air slowly and deeply. Swim. Do gentle range of motion exercises like bending forward, backward and sideways.

Nothing worthwhile comes quickly or easily. There is no such thing as a five-minute daily workout that will help you regain flexibility, stamina, strength and endurance. Your physical exercise program will require at least 30 minutes a day. It's important for you to perform these exercises while relaxed mentally. While you exercise, put other issues aside. Concentrate on breathing deeply and floating mentally in a tranquil sea.

The need to improve your life through physical exercise, therapy and rehabilitation cannot be overstated. The criterion of success? Measurably improved performance and function. When you become active and useful you are less prone to depression, chronic pain, despair, hopelessness and perpetual frustration. You cut the reverberating circuit.

Nine specific objectives and goals for an exercise program are:

1. Increased muscular strength

2. Increased muscular endurance

3. Increased flexibility

4. Increased blood flow to the muscles

5. Decreased muscular fatigue

6. Decreased muscular tightness

7. Decreased joint stiffness

8. Decreased inactivity

9. Decreased pain

Subduing the pain monster

Pain may be due to muscle tension or contraction. You can often control such pain by practicing simple stress management techniques. Deep breathing, progressive relaxation, biofeedback, self-hypnosis, yoga and swimming all relax, strengthen and stretch the muscles.

Yoga

Conceived as a way to integrate body, mind and spirit, yoga combines physical postures with good breathing. It is simple to perform and beneficial for the autonomic and central nervous systems. Yoga induces a natural state of meditation. It stretches and limbers the body and strengthens the muscle system. It brings you immediate body and breath awareness. In yoga, you assume and hold a position while you probe for pain spots and respond to them. Gradually, you overcome all tension and stiffness. Yoga keeps your body strong and ultimately benefits the original afflicted pain spot.

Swimming

Swimming rhythmically, with its concentration on breathing

and isolation from outside distractions, has similar benefits. The water is a world where you can be alone and tune in to yourself. The joint movements in swimming combat pain that has crept into your system, pain that has sucked life from your neck, back, shoulders, knees and hands. Because you are near weightless in the water, your joints work much more smoothly and effortlessly.

Almost any physical motion can be done in water, because the buoyancy of water supports weak and painful limbs. Water offers a gentle, definite resistance but can accommodate force when you expand and stretch your joints. While you swim, your tendons and ligaments stretch evenly and smoothly, increasing range of movement and strength. Swimming is a wonderful way to lose weight and relieve pressure on your back. Swimming will retard the aging process of your cardiovascular system.

Besides walking, yoga and swimming, another important exercise is strengthening your abdominal muscles. This takes perseverance. Nobody enjoys doing stomach exercises. But it is especially important if you have chronic low back pain. Make your stomach muscles stronger and you relieve some low back pain. The abdominal muscles can absorb some of the load from the lower back.

Here are some guidelines for your physical exercise program:

1. Set reasonable, task-oriented goals and stick to them, regardless of your pain. Performance here is not pain related, but goal related.

2. Master one task before you move on to another.

Exercise:

1. To relax upper body tension: Stand erect with feet apart and hands behind your neck. Bend the upper portion of your

body sideways, first to your right and hold for five seconds, then to your left for five seconds. Repeat several times.

2. To relax head, neck and shoulder muscles: Lie on your back, either on the floor or on an exercise pad. Tuck your hands under the small of your back, palms down. While lifting your head, shoulders and elbows off the floor, tighten your abdominal muscles. Hold for a count of five seconds, then lower. Repeat several times.

3. To relax back and thigh muscles: Lie on your back, flex your knees and place a small pillow under your neck. Take a deep breath and fully expand your chest. Now breathe out slowly. Repeat.

These three exercises can be done at home. Perform your exercises on a firm, comfortable surface and do them in the same place each day. Begin with a brief relaxation exercise. Perform each exercise slowly and smoothly. Remember, the mild stiffness or soreness you feel after you first exercise will disappear in three or four days. No special equipment is needed other than a floor exercise mat, a pillow and a towel. Optional equipment for more advanced exercise include a stationary bicycle and wall pulleys. I encourage you to do a variety of physical activities daily around your home: walking, swimming, gardening and, most importantly, stretching.

You will become more functional as you focus on productive activities instead of your pain. The key to beneficial exercise is to approach—but not hit—your working-to-tolerance level. Go beyond that and you trigger pain, which causes you to stop exercising because you fear more pain.

Quota system

Work toward a specific goal or "quota." No longer use bodily sensations or pain as your cue to stop. As Jim learned, a quota system is an effective way to increase your activity level and reduce your functional limitations. As Jim substituted activity for inactivity, he experienced less pain and more mobility. Initial quotas are set to make sure you win. No matter how easy it seems, never work beyond your assigned quota.

Record all your exercise performances. Logging your activities demonstrates that you successfully completed your physical exercise quota. You take control of your physical exercise program and monitor it. Your physical exercises are determined by you, not by changes in pain.

Gradually increase the amount of exercise. Don't stop due to pain, weakness or fatigue. Don't let chronic pain control your activity and behavior. Move at a pace that promises success.

Your self-imposed quota system should provide for rest immediately following your physical exercise. Your rest periods must follow a schedule and occur only after you have met your quota. Soon, with consistent progress, you'll automatically rest after completing your quota and noting your performance. Your exercise program should overcome your chronic pain, increase your mobility, strengthen your muscles and change moving and posture habits that might aggravate pain. The goal? To make smooth, relaxed movement habitual and to regain the comfortable use of your body.

While Bill Cosby was a Navy physical therapist he helped a sailor restore motion to a paralyzed arm. His account of the miraculous event highlights the value of a therapist's support and encouragement. Physical therapists want you to get well and know from experience and conviction that what they teach can make you better. Their positive expectations are contagious. They make you expect to get better. That makes you want to work, and you do.

If you do not have a physical therapist, carefully follow the instructions in this chapter. Each successful step you make propels you onward.

Your family's participation is a must when designing your program, setting your goal and monitoring your performance. Mrs. Siroti's husband was key in making sure his wife succeeded at her physical exercise program. He monitored the exercises she performed and prepared hot and cold packs for her use before and after her intense physical exercises. The positive interaction between them during her program served as an important reinforcer of their relationship.

Keeping an activity diary

Logging your activities hourly not only shows you how much each day you sit, stand, walk, recline or exercise, but also shows associations between activity and what happens within your psyche or even within your family. It may reveal that you stopped exercising only after a family member accused you of exaggerating your pain, or after some other upsetting experience at work or at home. It would greatly help the accuracy of your activity journal if a family member or close friend who interacts with you daily also notes your activities in the journal. Such observations pinpoint the relationship between your activity and your emotions at any given time.

Your personal comments are hints to your progress. As you

review your entries you'll spot relationships between what's going on in your life and how you feel. Then you can start to deal with situations that precipitate your chronic pain. Note when you feel tired or are in discomfort so you can adjust your activity schedule accordingly—adding relaxation exercises to forestall fatigue, play periods for discomfort, and exercise breaks to avert tension.

Stay focused and remember your short-term and long-term goals. Mastering physical and mental techniques that control pain is essential, but by themselves they won't make you well. You must also pay attention to the quality of your life. To get more out of being well you need to be emotionally up and physically busy. But you won't be comfortable until you are at ease in your body.

Exercise: Do these exercises to feel more comfortable in your body.

1. Learn how to touch your body. Softly run your fingertips across your entire body. Feel each crevice, the smooth and rough, the curvatures. Feel your muscles and your fat. They are all OK; they make up part of you.

2. How is your interest in sex? Are you using your chronic pain to avoid it? Explore with your mate your sexual roles. Exploring your sexual self helps you explore your physical self and gets you in tune physiologically and emotionally.

3. What do you do for fun? Have you returned to the sports and hobbies you once enjoyed? Have you found any new ones? List the activities you enjoyed before your chronic pain. If you once enjoyed walking, swimming, gardening or stretching, try them again. Try anything that doesn't exacerbate your pain, and do it daily. What hobbies will put you in touch with others and get you away from the television set? List things you are interested in, like going to an art muse-

um or doing charitable work, that encourages group interaction. Then do them. Become involved! Involvement gives you new direction in life and propels you with motivation and an upbeat spontaneity.

4. Are you beginning to take care of others and yourself again? Are you more aware of others' needs? Are you more determined to make relationships trusting, rewarding and close? List people who are important to you, including family members, co-workers, neighbors and friends. Note a few characteristics of each. What do they like to do? What characteristics make them unique? Now think of ways you can help them with their interests or join them in an activity they enjoy. You'll be surprised how much satisfaction you gain from being involved in activities others enjoy.

5. What are you doing about your work responsibilities? Have you changed your career goals? Have you met any problems head-on?

6. What about your non-working hours? Have you assumed your share of the workload at home? Do you again enjoy adult responsibility and challenge?

Ask these questions of yourself regularly, and answer them honestly. If you don't like the picture they paint, you know how to change the behavioral patterns that keep you from the satisfying life you want. Note that I didn't say the perfect life, or the problem-free life. But a satisfying life is a rewarding and achievable goal.

Being assertive at work

A great deal of stress comes from the need to master an impossible job situation. My patients have shown me that physical stress and painful muscles are almost always present when work conditions are untenable.

Some people reason that if something at work isn't satisfactory and their stress increases their chronic pain, it must be their fault. Others feel they must stoically remain at a job regardless of how much pain they suffer until they conquer the job. To leave is a cop-out. Still others need the world to feel sorry for them. Unconsciously they set up impossible job conditions. Their pain is aggravated and everyone murmurs words of sympathy. They gain the reinforcers they want—sympathy and concern—but not the reinforcers they need to heal.

Being assertive at work requires certain interactive skills. First, you need to be focused. Think through your work goals, the steps you must take, and how to use your talents to the fullest. Next, think how you can control your anxieties and fears. Inappropriate emotional reactions interfere with work performance. Tension produces fatigue, irritability, poor judgment. Fear of a work situation may mean you avoid the very task necessary to get the job done—and you fail to achieve your work goal.

The ability to manage change is essential. We tend to view change as stressful, but change is not the problem. How we feel about change determines whether or not we welcome it. With change comes opportunity. There is little to be gained in denying change. At any time in your life, some forces are pushing for change and others are resisting it. You need to be able to analyze these forces and decide in which direction to proceed.

You cannot manage your chronic pain differently if you cannot change, for it is change that refreshes and rejuvenates you and enables you to seek out new perspectives.

Exercise: Write down these beliefs about how change can alleviate chronic pain:

•This book is an opportunity to increase my skill and knowledge about my chronic pain—the causes, how and why it exacerbates, and its effects on my life.

•It is only through change that I can make progress.

•No decrease in my chronic pain is achieved without change.

•I can become someone who welcomes change because it gives my life more meaning. Change can move me to a higher level of consciousness.

Learn to accept change more readily by cultivating an attitude of openness and seeking opportunities to change the routines of your life. This affords you new avenues for healing.

Relaxation techniques

Physical relaxation techniques are as important as mental relaxation techniques. You may think of physical relaxation as no action. However, you must take action to relieve the muscle tension. Slow, gradual contraction and stretching of certain muscles allows them to relax. In doing so, you interrupt the unconscious signals that cause muscles to tighten involuntarily. So by taking action, you relax completely.

Relaxation training is especially effective when pain is accompanied by a sudden and dramatic increase in anxiety and muscle tension. Relaxation training is not physical therapy. You're learning exercises that let you temporarily escape life's frenetic activity and concentrate on relieving body tension. This can be a major tool not only to relieve pain, but to promote a lifetime of well-being.

Physical therapists, family practice and osteopathic physicians, orthopedic and rehabilitation medicine specialists and chiropractors use a number of physical modalities to control chronic pain.

Debra

Debra successfully managed her chronic pain using several of these modalities. Debra had a great deal of pain and muscle spasticity in her neck, shoulders and both sides of her face. She was an excellent candidate for Trans Electrical Nerve Stimulation (TENS).

A TENS unit is a small apparatus, about the size of a Walkman. TENS relieves pain by using electrodes to issue a periodic pulsing sensation to nerves just under the skin in an area of pain and muscle spasticity. Up to four areas on your body can be stimulated simultaneously. And you control the pulse settings yourself.

You start with the lowest setting, and amplitude is increased until you feel a strong tingling from the electrodes. You determine the level of intensity that is most comfortable, and the TENS unit effectively controls the pain. Anyone can quickly become adept at this modality.

How does it work? It delivers communication from your pain to your brain through a small amount of electric current. Research has proven that endorphin levels are significantly higher after TENS treatment.

After breakfast Debra would spend five minutes setting up her TENS treatment. She would place one electrode to the left of her mid-cervical neck area and one to the right; she placed an electrode on the muscle of her right shoulder and one on the left. The stimulation box, worn at her waist, was hidden by her clothes. Debra found the impulse intensity that was most comfortable, and off to work she went! For six hours her device was

on, while she worked, while she meditated, while she did creative visualization and guided imagery. She envisioned the
TENS machine exciting "good" nerve impulses and extinguish-
ing "bad" ones. Often during the day she complimented herself
for being so skillful!

Often the muscles in Debra's neck and shoulders were tense
and spastic with a knotting pain. A second modality that Debra
used was ice packs applied for ten minutes three or four times
a day. This broke up the tension and spasticity. Ice slows the
transmission of pain impulses along the nerve pathways.

Medical studies demonstrate that cold alters electrical muscle activity and significantly diminishes muscle spasticity. Ice
does not have the two major drawbacks of heat: Ice penetrates the
body deeper than heat, and ice constricts blood vessels, thereby
decreasing the chance of internal bleeding.

Ice massage can be used as often as needed with no harmful side effects. It helps relieve neck and back pain, painful joints
and muscle strains. Because ice message can be uncomfortable
when you first use it, allow a period of adjustment.

Rubbing the ice gently around the painful area brought Debra
the desired results. Debra also applied her newly found skills in
creative visualization and imagery. She envisioned the ice literally breaking up the muscle spasticity; as the ice melted, so did
her tension and pain.

Heat is a third modality that controls chronic muscle pain,
tension and spasticity. We all know heat eases aching, painful
muscles and joints; you have probably taken a hot bath or shower to ease pain. Heat's effect on spastic and tense muscles is
quite similar to that of cold. Heat soothes these muscles and
allows gentle range-of-motion and stretching exercises. This
combination—heat and then stretching exercises—is remarkably

effective in relaxing striated skeletal musculature and increasing the extensibility of collagen tissue.

However, there are positive and negative aspects to heat therapy. Heat can be effective for dilating blood vessels and increasing the amount of painful lactates that can be carried from the pain site. Unfortunately, heat does not penetrate deep below the skin, and may cause increased bleeding in an injury.

Things to do at home using heat to alleviate pain:

•*Take a hot shower* and allow the water to penetrate deep into sore muscles.

•*Place a hot, wet towel on aching areas.*

•*Use heating pads* on your tense, aching areas. Be careful to maintain them at a low intensity level and alternate your skin contact every 15 minutes to prevent superficial skin burns.

•*Use a whirlpool.* Whirlpools and Jacuzzis are available for home use or can be found in most health clubs. Adjust the water jets and position sore, tense muscle areas a few inches from them. The temperature should never exceed 110 degrees, and therapy should never exceed 20 minutes at a time.

For maximum effect, ultrasound, diathermy and hubbard tanks must be performed by a professional. Several physical modalities must be performed by a professional, too: massage, traction, biofeedback and manipulation. Although still controversial among conservative medical practitioners, manipulation using either osteopathy or chiropractic is now widely accepted as a valid treatment for chronic pain.

Posture is important to chronic pain. Osteopathic physicians believe incorrect or faulty posture impinges on nerves that supply the spinal cord. Aside from the pain this produces, your internal organs are affected and, thus, your whole body. A reverberating circuit develops, with impinged nerves affecting organs, which affect your nervous system.

Osteopathy firmly holds that restricted joint movement has a negative effect on surrounding tissues, circulation and breathing. These doctors claim that misalignment of the spine interferes with proper breathing. I discuss osteopathy in detail because osteopathic philosophy centers on holistic medicine. From its beginning, osteopathy's founder, Dr. Andrew Still, believed that the "whole man in his environment must be considered."

Biofeedback

For thousands of years Oriental holy men claimed they could consciously control their internal body functions. Western scientists consistently scoffed at their claims, but in the mid 1960s biofeedback researchers proved that it is indeed possible to consciously control autonomic body responses. Biofeedback is a method of controlling the body processes that, without specific training, cannot be regulated voluntarily. Biofeedback should be done only under direct supervision of a trained therapist. For most people, buying biofeedback equipment is neither practical nor advisable.

Biofeedback mirrors meditation in principle, but is mechanical in form. It is a monitoring device that uses elaborate instrumentation to measure your stress and muscle spasm as you simultaneously measure your tension, subjective as your measure might be.

Biofeedback teaches you how to control your body's tension. With an instrument panel, you can see how your brain controls your body's movements. As you meditate and relax, you'll see stress and tension dissipate. One surface electrode carries information from your brain to the machine, another from your hands and feet to the monitoring device. Still another electrode is placed on an area of pain. As you relax through imagery, your awareness of this area increases and you consciously ease your muscle tension. You increase the circulation to and thus the temperature in the affected area by concentrating on the area, sending warmth to dissipate and melt the pain. As you enter a state of total relaxation, your pain decrease is indicated on the monitor.

Biofeedback instruments measure temperature and muscle activity. When you're afraid or anxious, your hands get cold. When you're tense, your muscles tighten. By having wires attached to your limbs, the biofeedback machine picks up electrical activity and spews out accurate data, providing persuasive evidence that the pain cycle (anxiety, tension, pain) can be brought under your control. Biofeedback is an excellent modality to teach you that you can handle stress and tension constructively.

Not everyone can afford a sophisticated biofeedback machine. But you can create your own inexpensive biofeedback program at home. Your first step is using creative visualization and imagery to relax. Once you find the image that relaxes you, send warmth to your painful muscle areas. Close your eyes, breathe slowly and deeply, and use your hands as your heat gauges. Place one finger on the pain. Use imagery to increase the circulation into that area by creating an area of warmth. Visualization and meditation quiet your brain and allow your body to relax long enough to hear your inner voice create warmth.

This exercise should continue for about 30 minutes. It not only relieves your pain, but can reduce your stress, tension and anxiety. The result is clear: You are your own messenger; the messenger is from within.

Acupuncture

The Chinese believe acupuncture improves the balance between Yin and Yang and therefore changes the flow of life forces within the body. They believe the force of life falls within 12 meridians, or areas, of the body. Inserting a slender needle into specific meridian points affects other areas of the body. Strong evidence exists that acupuncture stimulates the production of the body's built-in painkiller and thereby relieves pain.

An interesting experiment conducted by the Medical College of Virginia attempted to determine if there was a link between acupuncture and the production of endorphins. They administered mild electrical shocks to the teeth of 35 volunteers and measured how much electricity was necessary before the subjects indicated they felt pain. Then each subject was given acupuncture between the thumb and forefinger for pain relief. The subjects were again shocked. This time their pain threshold (the amount of electricity needed before they indicated pain) increased 27 percent. Obviously, acupuncture had activated the production of the body's built-in painkiller.

Individuals with chronic pain tend to be those who were always caught up in a whirlwind of activity. Previously you were superenergetic, with that breathless, rushed feeling. There was a sense of being in a frantic hurry to get things done. Naturally, you are impatient with the slow, steady, regular exercises that are fundamental to your recovery. You will find that once you begin to improve, you'll get very uptight about relaxing: instead of relaxing, you will find yourself worrying about how much time your relaxation takes.

The purpose of this program is to change your high-pressured, tense, frenetic approach to life, to change the very way you move and react toward life. When you feel yourself getting impatient, breathe deeply and start over. All of the aspects of your chronic pain program—relaxation, meditation, breathing, imagery, writing and the physical exercises—are rehabilitative. They not only make you well, they help keep you well; this is the idea behind preventive medicine. It should become a lifetime routine for you, regardless of whether you are experiencing pain or not.

*Challenge faulty dialogues such as,
"I'll never change now."
See change as an opportunity.*

Reconditioning Your Mind 12

Not all responses to pain are learned. Some pain is simply response to an activity, like engaging in rigorous range-of-motion exercises or getting burned. As the cause of pain subsides (normal range-of-motion is restored, the burn heals) the pain abates and is forgotten.

What you learn to call pain is dependent on how your mind interacts with nerve endings and your state of mind when this message reaches your brain.

By combining cognitive, behavioral and operant psychology, you can change your attitude and behavior toward pain. And you can do so while following a rigorous exercise program that reinforces your thinking. As you become more active and can perform more tasks, you challenge your negative thinking. Your "I can'ts" become "I cans." And the more you change your negative thinking, the more you do.

Chronic pain is intertwined with associated behaviors. A child learns just what behaviors will gain attention and other rewards. When young Theodore Roosevelt had asthma attacks on Sundays, he demonstrated a learned response: Illness on Sunday meant much-needed attention—perhaps a special daytrip to the country—from his neglectful father.

The first big steps toward improvement are understanding that health is related to attitude, and taking responsibility for your physical and emotional well-being. The flip side? Negative thinking encourages pain behaviors that keep you helpless and debilitated. Stop negative self-talk by literally telling yourself to stop. If you devise a quick, non-negotiable response, there is no time to think about it. You just do it. Silent conversations inside your head about your chronic pain can be altered.

Jim

As Jim progressed in our pain-relief program, he learned how to breathe deeply and say to himself, "I'm not a bad or helpless person or a victim because I have pain. I am a good person. I can make my life worthwhile and productive. I can be happy." Jim slowly broke the reverberating circuit by turning negative thoughts into positive ones.

Behavioral and cognitive theories give you full responsibility to substitute your destructive view of yourself with a more positive view. You may not realize you have acquired bad habits that make you think of yourself as an invalid. But constant grimaces, groans or nonstop complaints can and will damage relationships with fellow workers and family.

Cognitive therapy and behavioral and operant conditioning might appear to be short-term, but they are problem-solving approaches that will help you, even if you believe your problem is strictly physical. By using them, you take an assertive step to intercede in the thinking-feeling-acting mode we call "behavior." This step can be further reinforced with a successful physical exercise program.

This point is a transition from the concrete (physical) aspect of my program to the abstract (creative visualization, imagery, meditation). In this transition you learn to combine these two spheres to generate a flow of ideas to make your inner self stronger. The aim is to strengthen your self-image and sense of autonomy. Armed with new communication skills, you can better express your needs and feelings to those around you, despite the presence of chronic pain.

Cognitive therapy

Cognitive therapy trains your mind to interpret the outside world more positively. This therapy changes your perception of your situation from a glass half empty to a glass half full. If you see the sky as partly cloudy rather than partly sunny, your happiness quotient is probably low and your pain factor is high.

Train your mind to recognize your automatic verbal and pictorial thoughts. Learn to use your mind to counter emotion-laden feelings that exacerbate pain. Life is a process of change. Yet you may resist change, believing your pain will worsen with changes in your life. Such beliefs may stem from past experience or from the way you currently handle change. Analyze your feelings of resistance and seek out a trusted listener to hear your concerns. Challenge faulty dialogues such as "I'll never change now." See change as an opportunity.

You can direct change in the way you manage pain with these four steps:

1. Choose the right situations.

2. Prepare for these situations.

3. Behave assertively during these situations.

4. Review these situations afterward.

Behavioral changes come in small steps. If you start with a very difficult situation, you may take too big a first step. Failure now may reduce your confidence in your ability to be assertive.

The first of the above four steps is the most difficult. Choose situations in which you have a good chance of maintaining your change in behavior. Also consider the benefits and consequences that can follow from increased assertion. Look for situations where the potential benefits clearly outweigh the risks.

Step two, preparing for a situation, is crucial. If you spend time before an important situation mentally walking through step three, you are more likely to succeed at step three. Preparing gives you confidence, and you behave more assertively.

Finally, review your results realistically. Rationally analyze what happened, and learn from it. This is your chance to work on improved responses to the situation. And by gaining some success, you can choose to stand up to a more difficult situation next time.

Learning self-control skills increases self-reliance and independence. You acquire a new empowerment over your chronic pain. This enables you to replace depression/anxiety, resignation/pessimism with courage/self-appreciation, hope/optimism. You substitute new thoughts for the old. The foundation of cognitive theory is that your thoughts create your emotions. Your perception of a situation determines how you react to it.

By combining cognitive therapy with imagery, you alter the emotions associated with chronic pain. You form an image that is positive and uplifting.

Try it! Visualize your pain. For example, if you have neck pain, visualize a tightening band around your neck. If you suffer chronic low-back pain, imagine dull fragments piercing your lower back. Examine this image carefully. Focus on form, texture and appearance. As you do, you become increasingly comfortable with your pain.

Now apply cognitive therapy: Change the image to a more favorable one. Because the image has become familiar, it is no longer as threatening. You are changing it to something you can control. That jagged, blunt edge at your back becomes a red ribbon hanging loosely at your waist. The tightening band around your neck becomes a soft piece of fabric worn as a collar or scarf.

Once you can transform these images and develop a sense of control, you can proceed to the next step: Let your images dim and disappear. Open your eyes and feel, think and act differently about your chronic pain.

Operant conditioning and behavioral theory

Operant conditioning is what happens when you reward yourself for success. You can use behavioral and operant conditioning to reinforce and sustain your pain behavior, or to eliminate it through a reward and punishment system you create. Praise and attention for good behavior are usually the best rewards.

Clinical studies show that activity schedules and graded task assignments are effective in behavioral therapy because they produce conceptual changes. Behavioral therapy is primarily concerned with your actions: You are directed to be more active and assertive, taking charge of your situation.

When you add cognitive therapy to expose and correct your negative distortions of these activities, you have synergized the two theories. To cope with chronic pain, the assigned tasks are setting specific goals, planning work and social activities, and becoming engrossed in your physical exercise program. These activities keep your mind off your pain.

Chapter 8 discussed medication reduction. When I discussed taking medication on a time-contingent rather than symptom-contingent basis, I utilized a key principle of operant conditioning: Reinforce well behavior. You learn to manage your chronic pain by eliminating drug dependence, dealing with your underlying depression, improving your family and community support systems and attaining goals that increase your quality of life.

Where to start

Once you and your family decide you are ready, as a group, for change, pinpoint behaviors or activities each of you will change.

Margot

Margot's initial challenge was to get out of bed more and do some physical activities—useful tasks such as setting the table or doing small household tasks that allowed her to fully range her painful joints. She logged five physical activities per day, enabling her to see how much progress she made on a daily basis.

At the end of each day, Margot wrote down how she felt, how her joints felt and whether her endurance and muscle strength had increased. Margot's husband had his own challenge: to attend less to her every request and do more for himself—for instance, resuming his Saturday golf games.

Having determined behaviors you think will work, you want to use reinforcers—attention, praise, solitude, serenity—consistently. Margot's husband felt guilt-stricken every time he ignored his wife's complaints of pain. But he persisted in attending her less, while praising her slightest effort to do things on her own. The result? Margot stopped complaining and became more active. The operant stimulus was now focused on Margot's well behavior, such as her increased endurance, muscle strength and ability to accomplish daily tasks. Her rewards were feeling better and her husband's attention, which she now received only when she exhibited well behavior.

Alvin

Acquiring new behaviors can mean survival at work. Alvin, another patient, was so preoccupied with his condition that he made no effort to relate to his co-workers. Overwhelmed by his chronic pain and believing there was no hope, he only frowned and grimaced, alienating himself from everyone.

The multi-disciplinary center staff made Alvin aware of what he was doing. Alvin said he was unaware of his body language, but he worked on it. He learned to say "no" to grimacing and frowning. He learned to make eye contact, smile and pay attention while talking with colleagues. This made an enormous difference in Alvin's progress with his co-workers.

Team members at the center taught Alvin how to view his work environment as a friendly one. He was encouraged to think of it as a place to build skills and friendships. A formerly negative environment became a more pleasing one. Interacting with friends helped Alvin focus less and less on back and leg pain.

Replacing pain-oriented attitudes and behaviors with healthy ones feels better than being guilty, blaming yourself and assuming the role of victim. You take responsibility, which confirms your ability to change and validates your power. Your inner being becomes a magnificent guide. The subtle reality that underlies our apparent reality encompasses our physical, emotional, mental and spiritual essence. In the next chapter, you will learn how to tap those powers more directly.

Take chances:
You will succeed only if you are fearless of failure.

When Things Fail 13

Controlling your pain is not easy. The path is beset by road-blocks. You may take two steps forward and one step back. But perceived failures are opportunities for growth. Take chances: You will succeed only if you are fearless of failure. Convert your energy into visions of success. My pain relief program is a process, not something you accomplish in a New York minute!

Imagine that you are climbing a high mountain; ascending that path sometimes entails taking downhill traverses. The same is true in your path to recovery. You are pleased with your progress. However, as you face the next step, you see the obstacle ahead. It might be a tough one: Looking for work that doesn't exacerbate your pain. Making a change in your life choices. Choosing activities rather than escaping into drugs and alcohol when you are confronted with tough problems. Feeling stressed and anxious is normal. If you expect these crises along the way, you will overcome them and keep going.

When your chronic pain knocks you down, get up. No matter how many times you are felled by your pain, keep getting up. As you enter the grays and blues of your feelings you have the golden opportunity to change your life.

Push yourself to do the exercises in this book. Take creative visualization, imagery or meditation exercises to the edge. When you think you are done, go further. That is often when you receive a strong message from the deep recesses of your mind. The prospect of losing control might be frightening, but you can come out stronger and more fulfilled.

A part of you may be afraid to heal your chronic pain, because with success you must give up your sorrows, misfortunes and righteous indignation, and tackle the world on a new footing. You must claim a higher purpose for your life, and that means change and a great deal of effort. But the time has come to heal. Wake up to the power that resides within you and leave behind life's pettiness.

Exercise: Wake up!

1. In your notebook list all the things you wish to accomplish but have not attempted—due to pain.

2. Write down why, in fact, you are now able to attempt them.

3. Envision yourself cheering on your success rather than rationalizing your excuses.

Make three big promises to yourself:

1. I will not limit my ability to succeed.

2. I will not wallow in my failures.

3. I can reach deeper within myself to heal my pain.

When the task seems impossible, tap into your spiritual self. You can do it! Chronic pain is physical, mental and spiritual. Help in the spiritual sphere is what you need when you fail. It's the fuel you need to begin again. You may wonder how you can be restored to health by beliefs, but the spiritual life is not theory. It is alive—you have to practice and live it each day.

Fear is a serious obstacle to your recovery. Pain has put you out of commission physically, mentally and emotionally. You have accommodated to pain by gradually becoming nothing. Fear is a by-product of the helplessness you've learned from pain. You are so immobilized and paralyzed that the slightest challenge to your inertia is frightening. You have lost control. As a consequence you have lost confidence in yourself and your ability to move at all. You know you must move onward, but the unknown is overwhelming.

You are afraid to face the responsibility of marriage, sex, family and career that comes with recovery. You may fear ever being a responsible person again. Anticipate these fears and they're easier to cope with. They're normal and transient. It is reassuring to know that they will abate with your first move.

In this chapter, forgiveness is the key. Forgive yourself for perceived failures, then move on. Once you forgive yourself, you'll no longer fear practicing this chronic pain control program. You are dealing head-on with your fear of failure. You can confront the past. Once you forgive yourself for perceived failures—like being addicted to medication or alcohol—you are ready to understand how to overcome your pain.

Debra

Debra learned to forgive herself for feeling anxious at work. Jim learned to forgive himself for lying in bed, drinking, and withdrawing from life. And Laura forgave herself for blaming herself for the sexual abuse she suffered as a child. By forgiving yourself you are ready for a new beginning. Simply put, forgiveness is peace. Forgiving yourself signals self-healing.

Exercise: Here are six forgiveness exercises:

1. Every morning make a conscious decision to combat your chronic pain.

2. Upon awakening, plan the day you want to have. Convince yourself, by repeating several of the affirmations in this book, that this day can happen exactly as you wish.

3. Throughout the day, take time for quiet reflection. We get caught up in events and don't take time for our inner selves. Even if you just sit where you are, take time out for quiet reflection and re-experience the inner you. Visualize the feelings you wish to have and the activities you wish to experience.

4. Every time you provoke attack against yourself, stop. Take quick, restorative, forgiving action. Remember the day you want to have, how you want to control the pain, and what has occurred that is not part of that plan. A change in your reaction pattern enables you to transform calamity into serenity. Repeat several times: "I have another way to look at my chronic pain. I now look at life differently."

5. Agree not to judge yourself or your reactions to situations as they arise. Don't be concerned if you are not successful in resolving your chronic pain problem each and every time. If you become overly concerned, you'll find that fear arises and you'll attack yourself for any perceived failures.

6. Keep your mind open to infinite possibilities. Keep the image of Jim in your mind. He regained control over his life by exercising and repeating positive messages to himself. In the beginning of his recovery, he wanted to replace inactivity with action. He saw himself returning to work, playing with his children, enjoying sex with his wife. He repeated this image long before it was a reality. This is how Jim wanted to live. Eventually, he did just that.

What you can learn is limitless, because your mind is limitless. As an affirmation, continuously remind yourself: "I have limitless awareness and creative powers."

Failure, then, is the failure to do, to understand, to learn anew. By trying again, you will succeed. You cannot heal through fear. Misery is the longest road to joy.

You are off to create a new life for yourself—one with new insights from your inner spirit. Your strength lies in joy, not pain. As you find increasing joy and harmony in your life, you have less and less tolerance for hiding behind your pain.

Following a program of physical therapy, meditation, creative visualization, imaging and responsibility is far more difficult than taking pills, having multiple surgeries and blaming others. Ignore temporary setbacks. Renew your efforts. Commend yourself for the progress you make.

When things do fail, these exercises can show you how success builds on itself.

Exercise: Go back in your memory and relive a previously successful experience. Remember how your participation sparked that success. Let your mind fill in every detail. The more detail the better. By remembering what happened when you were successful, you recreate the entire event.

Perhaps you remember when you knitted that beautiful sweater for your daughter, the time you built that handy kitchen cabinet, the time you installed the garage door opener much to your neighbors' amazement. Imagine feeling exactly like you felt then. Because self-confidence builds on past successes, your vivid memories are strengthening your success thought patterns.

You are a responsible individual rather than a helpless and hopeless victim.

Exercise: A self-fulfilled individual nourishes his or her self-respect. Learn to see yourself as able and self-reliant, possessing a mastery over your chronic pain. As you program yourself for success, concentrate on building confidence, self-esteem and self-expression. Visualize your past successes over your chronic pain time after time.

Debra is an excellent example of this point. She became a true pro at meditation, creative visualization and guided imagery. She was duly proud of her success in mastering these techniques and continuously reinforced this success.

Visualize your success at the exercises discussed in previous chapters. Recall how those exercises eventually helped relieve some of your wrenching pain. Congratulate yourself on your increased range of motion.

Recall your success at visualization, your ability to create that gently flowing brook, the acres of roses, the magic of the ocean's waves, the brilliant snow-capped mountains. Rise above your perceived failures as you reach the dignity of self-fulfillment.

Express your success. It's your right to feel good about yourself. In fact, you can feel good about yourself even when you make mistakes and fail. The best basketball star misses many shots. Does he feel like a failure? No. He feels great knowing that more often he helps propel his team to victory.

You can learn from your mistakes and failures. What's important is that you get up again, start anew, follow the suggestions in this book. Remember those times when you tried again, no matter how difficult, and came out a survivor.

Because you will occasionally fail to reach your goal of pain control, learn to tolerate a certain degree of frustration without becoming upset. We all learn a great deal from our mistakes.

You have suffered enough. Now it's time for you to move forward. Use a mind-body-spirit approach—like meditation—to withdraw from the world of pain and ponder what's going on in your life. Do what Debra did: Remove yourself from your frenetic workday environment by mentally placing yourself at the beach. Stare at the magnificence of the ocean. Train your unconscious mind to tell you that your essential goodness is unchangeable. It is what we say to ourselves that counts. As Jean Paul Sartre stated: "Man was nothing much other than what he made of himself."

How you interpret the world around you and how you interpret your pain are your choices. Your mind can see whatever you want it to see. The power over your mind is yours. Use that power to create a world of productivity and greatness. Medical scientists believe man uses only a small portion of his mental capabilities. Stretch that use. Encompass an entire new world of perception.

You respond to what you perceive. If it is your core belief that you will fail to control your pain, then you will perceive yourself as a failure. Yes, acknowledge your weakness. Then do something about it! When you transcend your body's boundaries, you transcend all limitations. What you are is what you think you are. Don't think of yourself as a failure.

Mrs. Siroti

Mrs. Siroti was unable to walk just a few blocks to the chronic pain center. Once she was engaged in our approach, she envisioned herself walking those few blocks. She saw herself taking each step, a self-reliant and independent woman. Eventually she didn't need to depend on her husband, and came to the center on her own.

Like so many of the patients at the multi-disciplinary center, you can deal with your chronic pain. Quiet introspection and meditation permit you to rise above daily strife and evaluate your priorities. But your pain might be stubborn. It's not going to disappear overnight. Patterns take time to develop; they take time to break.

Recovery will be your story of success. You will accept a new life. You will have new experiences. Recovering from the grips of chronic pain is like being reborn. Acknowledge to yourself that recovery is a process. It's something you'll always work on. Your keys to success are passion, persistence, truth, trust, clarity and growth.

Exercise: Try an exercise I use for patients engulfed in failure. This exercise emphasizes that recovery is a process. Whether you use creative visualization, meditation, breathing, yoga or imaging to control your pain, the stages and procedures are:

1. **Orientation.** Point out the problem: "I have chronic pain of the (identify the pain site). I am addicted to specific pain medications and tranquilizers."

2. **Preparation.** Gather pertinent data, such as the time of the day your pain appears or what precipitates it: "I have pain in the morning/afternoon/evening. I have pain following activity/inactivity. I have pain when I sit/stand. I have pain when I'm feeling anxious and nervous/when the kids are out of control."

As Debra realized, feeling pain when you feel anxious is not unusual. Whenever she felt particularly anxious at work, Debra noticed that the pain in her jaws, face and cervical neck became exceptionally bothersome.

Gathering your pertinent pain data might reveal other problems, as my patient Marc discovered. "I have a drug problem; I am addicted to pain drugs and tranquilizers. I take these drugs whenever I feel anxious, tired or in pain."

3. **Ideation.** Identify alternatives by envisioning ideas and turning them into statements you repeat to yourself several times a day:

A. "Instead of focusing on my failures, I can meditate, do mental relaxation exercises like creative visualization and imagery, or perform lower back and neck exercises, along with general physical exercises."

B. "Instead of suppressing my anger and letting it fester and travel to my lower back, I can call somebody in my chronic pain support group and share these feelings."

C. "Instead of repressing my feelings over various situations in nonproductive and unhealthy ways, I can release these feelings by writing them down."

D. "Instead of focusing on my pain and letting it interfere with my marriage, I'll try those new communication skills."

E. "Instead of heaping a handful of pills into my body and tuning out the world, I'll try relaxation and stretching exercises."

4. **Incubation.** Invite illumination. Go with the flow. It helps you move upward and onward. Once my patients see the light, they travel to places they thought they could never go. They triumph over their pain and reach a higher level of consciousness. Focus on your internal state. Quiet your mind so you'll acquire a vision.

5. **Evaluation.** Judge your new ideas:

   A. Are my ideas working? Do I focus on the unlimited possibilities rather than on my mistakes and failures?

   B. Have I learned to trust my subconscious and unconscious?

   C. Am I focusing on my work?

   D. Am I beginning to see my world differently?

   E. Am I willing to struggle and try again to get my new ideas implemented?

   F. Am I taking ideas from my unconscious and putting them into action?

6. **Execution.** See if the idea works:

   "Am I making progress step-by-step? Am I less dependent, less addicted to drugs? Am I communicating and interacting better with my family and others? I understand that this is a process. Do I understand that overcoming the fear of failure is the key? Am I pushing through the fear barriers? Do I believe that something in my true self—in my core being—will let me triumph over my pain?"

Let's review exercises to do when things fail:

1. Know your direction.

2. Remind yourself that your goal is control of your chronic pain.

3. Understand your commitment. Make strong choices about your desire to heal your pain. Make up your mind that this is the path you are going to follow. Show conviction.

4. Compile the information necessary, including the resources available to you to combat pain.

5. Have the courage to act. Only by actions can your pain control become a reality.

6. Develop a genuine interest in and respect for others. By reaching out to others—family, co-workers, friends—you become involved. By engaging in discussion groups, you become charitable toward others. You'll soon realize how easy it is to be charitable with yourself.

7. Assume responsibility for your pain. Take charge of your situation. Appreciation of your own inner worth musters up greater self-esteem.

8. Use assertive techniques in everyday situations. Then extend them to more important things, like your inner feelings toward people around you.

9. Increase your confidence at assuming control by remembering your past successes.

10. Practice affirmations and focus on positive thoughts to achieve positive results. Continuously feed these positive thoughts into you conscious and unconscious mind. Repetition and persistence are the key.

The art of self-acceptance is your next exercise. Come to terms with your progress, whatever it might be. Failures in your program belong to you, but are not you. You make mistakes, but you are not the mistake. Separate your actions from your being. It's important to tolerate imperfection and accept yourself.

Barbara

When Barbara entered our multi-disciplinary chronic pain center, she was eager to deal with her physical pain. After two months as a patient, she learned how emotional and psychological elements influenced her physical pain. But it was only after she examined her spiritual life that the whole picture became clear. Using the techniques of relaxation, meditation and creative visualization, Barbara reached a clear state of serenity. From there she could re-direct her life and formulate new priorities. An awareness of a power greater than yourself is the essence of the spiritual.

When you do something to change the direction of your life, you become assertive with your life. This empowers you with tremendous energy.

In the traditional medical model, the physician reinforces your dependency and your belief in magical cures. In the traditional model, we emphasize the physician's responsibility to us rather than our responsibility to ourselves.

It may be hard to see how far you've traveled, because recovery happens slowly, step-by-step. You proceed by accomplishing sub-goals. To get an idea of whether your new way of thinking, feeling and behaving works, retake the Attitude Questionnaire in Chapter 6. You should see significant changes. Any negative answers that remain negative are your next challenge. In a year, if you take the questionnaire again, you will be amazed by your transformation.

After retaking the Attitude Questionnaire, consider these five additional questions:

1. Do I fall short of my dreams and goals in controlling my pain?

2. Do I focus too much on past mistakes and failures?

3. Do I feel empty?

4. Am I afraid of rejection?

5. Am I afraid to let others know me because they will then know who I really am?

Carefully dissect your answers. How do your perceived failures influence your answers to these questions? Listen to yourself. Learn about yourself. Consider how your answers are influenced by: fear, resentment, anger, envy, guilt, forgiveness, patience, humility, peacefulness and tranquility.

How dominant are the first five emotions (fear, resentment, anger, envy, guilt)? How about the second five (forgiveness, patience, humility, peacefulness, tranquility)? How can you shift your focus away from the first five and toward the second five? Make this a primary goal in your chronic pain control program.

The more you get in touch with your reality, including your pain, the more you will accept, without judgment, the way things are. You have trained your mind to repress things. By carefully listening, you can become a mirror that reflects the reality that is around you.

The multi-dimensional mind-body-spirit program works, and works well! You can reach your goal if you pursue it. Along the way, be compassionate with yourself, your family and others who share your odyssey. By touching your inner selves and welcoming life, you give each other the most precious gift anyone can bestow.

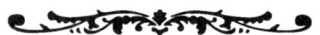

Remember, the only time you fail
is when you make the choice to quit.

Caring for Yourself

14

The goal in recovery is to become a self-fulfilled individual with nourished self respect. You want to appear in your own eyes as likable, wanted, accepted and able. You now possess the information and knowledge necessary to control your chronic pain. More importantly, you are self-reliant and responsible, full of self-esteem and self-respect. You know how to release your own energy, freeing yourself from a self-imposed prison of pain.

You can find help and resources for your journey wherever you are. You can combine services available at the Veterans Administration, community hospitals, physical therapy clinics, outreach facilities, community mental health centers, social service agencies and libraries. You can set up your own unique pain management program.

If you do not live near a multi-disciplinary chronic pain facility or a similar musculoskeletal rehabilitation center, it is possible to rehabilitate yourself at home. This includes exercises to regain full strength, range of motion and endurance. They must be pain-free and performed smoothly, with no limping, twitching or other abnormal response. They must be progressive—that is, progressively more complex and challenging without pain. Movements should be undertaken slowly and the range of movement should stay well within comfortable limits. In time, you can perform more exercises and increase your mobility and range of movement. Your exercises should focus on regaining normal joint motion, muscular strength, endurance and speed.

You regain range of motion with stretching exercises and repetitive motions. In stretching exercises, move the involved joint and/or muscle to its limit of motion and hold the position for 30-60 seconds. As your muscles relax, adjust the position just enough to maintain the stretch over 30-60 seconds. Repeat over the next several days. You can regain a greater range of motion by moving your musculature through the available range of motion repetitively. Your goal is to stretch any contractures, reduce adhesions and restore mobility to your joints. Perform the physical exercises only until you begin to feel pain; make no attempt to stretch beyond that point of mobility.

As you do these exercises, practice your breathing. Feel your ribs rising and your abdomen protruding slightly as your diaphragm contracts when you inhale. Exhale deeply and slowly, allowing your ribs to move lower as you pull in your abdomen. Relax for several seconds and perform your stretching exercises again, using the same breathing technique.

Inactivity aggravates pain; physical exercise helps you heal. When you combine physical exercise, deep breathing and mental exercises (meditation, creative visualization, imagery and relaxation), you restore yourself and promote healing.

In addition, these physical and breathing exercises have far-reaching effects on your cardiovascular and metabolic systems, further aiding your healing.

Cool your areas of chronic pain at home with ice immersion or ice massage for 15-20 minutes to partially numb the area. Then exercise again, without crossing the pain limits. Ice again, this time for five minutes, and exercise for another five minutes. Repeat these five-minute cycles three more times.

As you regain your range of motion, you can also build muscle strength. I'm not talking about lifting heavy free weights. I am suggesting isotonic exercises using small weights, and flexion and extension exercises.

Be assertive in these exercises! Access the resources in your community for chronic pain patients. If your community does not have specific programs, use community groups and direct-service agencies. Mobilize support for your needs within a direct-service agency by linking various other community groups and organizations. This becomes part of your communication and socialization network, and helps you integrate pain management with the rest of your life.

You have learned how to network and participate in social support groups and systems. You can implement a plan to create a coordinated treatment system for yourself within your community. You can find a local general practitioner skilled at osteopathic manipulation, eliminating the need to travel to an in-patient referral treatment center.

To take back control of your life, you have to return to work. Work helps define you, and provides you with essential self-esteem and a sense of self-accomplishment. Work challenges your mind and body. It stimulates you, makes you feel capable and confident. Start thinking about what you have done, what you want to do and what you can reasonably expect to do again. Plan for and move toward a work goal at the very start of your program.

You need to restore a sense of mastery over your life. The illusion that someone will take care of you is just that: illusion.

Life offers no free rides! It hurts to be helpless and dependent. When you are robbed of your independence, you are robbed of yourself. That's what the invalidism of chronic pain does to you. The only way to move onward with chronic pain is to help yourself. Look inside, not to others. That's where your pain-free future begins!

It takes perseverance and diligence, but as long as you stay with it, you will succeed. Remember, the only time you fail is when you make the choice to quit. Just give it all of your hope and desire. Be patient, and hold on to your vision.

About the Author

Dr. Claude Amarnick (1947-1995) founded several leading chronic pain management centers in New York, Florida and California. As the director of a much-heralded chronic pain facility in Burbank, Cal., Dr. Amarnick appeared as an expert on a week-long NBC television series on chronic pain. His strategies to combat chronic pain are utilized by many medical facilities throughout the United States, and have helped thousands of Americans escape pain.

Dr. Amarnick received a bachelor's degree in 1969 from the University of Pennsylvania, and graduated from the Philadelphia College of Osteopathic Medicine in 1973. He completed his residency in physical and rehabilitation medicine at the University of Pennsylvania, and was board certified in this specialty. He completed a second residency in psychiatry at the U.C.L.A. Medical Center and at the Beth Israel Medical Center in New York, and was board eligible in this specialty.

Dr. Amarnick served on the medical staff and faculty at the Mount Sinai Medical School in New York, where he lectured on the psychiatric implications of various physical disabilities, including chronic pain. He developed a reputation among his peers as a expert in chronic pain, lecturing to various medical groups, hospital staffs and medical conferences, including a national conference of rehabilitation medicine specialists.

Dr. Amarnick is the author of several books and numerous professional articles, which continue to be published posthumously in medical journals worldwide. Garrett Publishing will publish a second book by Dr. Amarnick this year, addressing how to keep our aging Americans out of nursing homes. Dr. Amarnick's published articles include:

"Sexual Abuse & Healing Chronic Pelvic Pain,"
Alternative Medical Journal, Nov./Dec. 1994

"Exercise and the Elderly," "The Real Meaning of Relaxation,"
Alternative Medical Journal, Jan./Feb. 1995

"The Folk High School," Inner Self, April 1995

"Spirituality Through Folk High School,"
Townsend Letter for Doctors, April 1995

"Quest for the Spirit,"
Alternative Medical Journal, May/June 1995

"Sexual Abuse and Pelvic Pain,"
Journal of Alternative and Complementary Medicine, July 1995

"Growing Old is O.K.," Explore More, Aug. 1995

"How You Can Offer a Helping Hand When Signs of Alcoholism Mirror the Aging Process,"
Townsend Letter for Doctors, Aug./Sept. 1995

"Old Should Not Mean Idle,"
Journal of Alternative and Complementary Medicine, October 1995

Index